Practical Issues in Geriatrics

Series Editor

Stefania Maggi
Aging Branch
CNR-Neuroscience Institute
Padua
Italy

This practically oriented series presents state of the art knowledge on the principal diseases encountered in older persons and addresses all aspects of management, including current multidisciplinary diagnostic and therapeutic approaches. It is intended as an educational tool that will enhance the everyday clinical practice of both young geriatricians and residents and also assist other specialists who deal with aged patients. Each volume is designed to provide comprehensive information on the topic that it covers, and whenever appropriate the text is complemented by additional material of high educational and practical value, including informative video-clips, standardized diagnostic flow charts and descriptive clinical cases. Practical Issues in Geriatrics will be of value to the scientific and professional community worldwide, improving understanding of the many clinical and social issues in Geriatrics and assisting in the delivery of optimal clinical care.

More information about this series at http://www.springer.com/series/15090

Bernard Swynghedauw

The Biology of Senescence

A Translational Approach

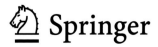 Springer

Bernard Swynghedauw
French Institute of Health and Medical Research
Paris
France

ISSN 2509-6060   ISSN 2509-6079   (electronic)
Practical Issues in Geriatrics
ISBN 978-3-030-15110-2   ISBN 978-3-030-15111-9   (eBook)
https://doi.org/10.1007/978-3-030-15111-9

This Springer imprint is published by the registered company Springer Nature Switzerland AG
The registered company address is: Gewerbestrasse 11, 6330 Cham, Switzerland

Acknowledgment

Firstly, the author wishes to give many thanks to his wife for her patience during what has been the fairly arduous writing of this book. He must also give his warm thanks to Professor Patrick Assayag who founded the special course on cardiovascular geriatric medicine in Kremlin-Bicêtre Hospital (Paris University) and who helped him so much in the conception and production of this book. Many thanks also go to Professors Raymond Ardaillou and Yvan Touitou from the French *Académie de Médecine*, Professors Bernard Levy and Sophie Besse, and Drs. Gaele Aubert and Serge Rabenou for providing clever and friendly advices and also to Rodgers Hickman for helping in correcting his English.

The author is a Clinician and a Former Teacher who directed a laboratory of biomedical research for many years, which focused on the molecular and evolutionary cardiology and also the nonlinear analysis of heart rate variability. As such, he is fully aware that biomedical language is not easy for clinicians. It is frequent that clinicians, when seated next to their patients, feel that complexity is their "privilege"; they should also realize that biology is now progressively approaching a true representation of the complexity of life.

Abbreviations

AD	Alzheimer's disease
AGE	Advanced glycation end products
AGSMRCV	Age-standardized mortality rate for CV disease
AIDS	Acquired immune deficiency syndrome
AGE	Advanced glycation end products
CNTD	Chronic nontransmissible diseases
COPD	Chronic obstructive pulmonary disease
CR	Calorie restriction
CryAB	Alpha B-crystallin, also called HSPB5
CV	Cardiovascular
DALYS	Disability-adjusted life years
DHA	Docosahexaenoic acid
DCM	Diabetic cardiomyopathy
ECM	Extracellular matrix
GBDS	Global burden of disease study
GDP	Gross domestic product
HLE	Healthy life expectancy
HF	Heart failure
HFpEF	Heart failure with preserved ejection fraction
HCSP	*Haut Conseil de la Santé Publique*
HSP	Heat-shock proteins
IL	Interleukin
INCa	*Institut National du Cancer*
IPF	Idiopathic pulmonary fibrosis
INSERM	*Institut National de la Santé et de la Recherche Médicale*
IPCC	Intergovernmental Panel on Climate Change
LDL	Low-density lipoproteins
LV	Left ventricle
Mb	Megabase
miR	Micro-ribonucleic acids
MRI	Magnetic resonance imaging
mRNA	Messenger ribonucleic acid
NAT	*N*-acetyltransferase
NF-kappa B	Nuclear factor-kappa B

NMR	Nuclear magnetic resonance
NSPC	Neural stem/progenitor cells
PET	Photon emission computed tomography
PGC	Peroxisome proliferator-activated receptor coactivator gamma
ROS	Reactive oxygen species
SASP	Senescence-associated secretory phenotype
SC(s)	Senescent cell(s)
SPECT	Single-photon emission computed tomography
TGF	Tumor growth factor
TNF	Tumor necrosis factor
TLR	Toll-like receptor
VEGF	Vascular endothelial growth factor

Contents

Introduction

Abstract

Ageing is the time-dependent functional decline that affects a living species. Senescence is as complicated as life. The mean lifespan of humans has been increasing for a century and population ageing has shaped a totally new medical landscape.

Ageing, "the time-dependent functional decline that affects most living species" [1] is associated with the gradual accumulation of a variety of cellular and molecular damage, which, over time, leads to reduced physiological reserves and an increased risk of several chronic diseases, this is the definition of ageing for the World Report on Ageing and Health from the World Health Organization in 2015. The biology of ageing is a complicated issue, just like the biology of life.

The mean human lifespan has been increasing for roughly a century, even if it appears to be reaching a limit (see the Preface of JF Toussaint in [2]). The risk of dying increases with age, but a model published recently by an Italian group predicts that this trend flattens out after 105 years [3, 4]. Population ageing has shaped a totally new medical landscape [5–7] and is becoming a crucial problem for public health economies [8–11].

It would be presumptuous to offer a simple solution to such a fast-changing topic. Nevertheless, there is, for the moment at least, one line of approach which provides consistent and consensual solutions to the clinical landscape. In the following text, we shall limit our statement to findings that have clinical applications or, at least, provide clinicians with a fairly simple biological explanation of their current practices.

The biology of senescence is likely to be as complicated as the biology of life (Table 1.1)—which should no longer be a surprise to anyone, and this book simply aims to focus on the question in 2018 with, as a guiding thread, the one proposed by the Mayo Clinic group of van Deursen [13–18], and adopted by many other authors

© Springer Nature Switzerland AG 2019   1
B. Swynghedauw, *The Biology of Senescence*, Practical Issues in Geriatrics,
https://doi.org/10.1007/978-3-030-15111-9_1

Table 1.1 The definition of life

For Koshland [12], the past editor-in-chief of *Science*, there is no simple definition of life, like, for example, the ability to reproduce. Life also exists in the absence of reproduction, and to define life, it is desirable to elucidate its essential thermodynamic and kinetic principles. He proposed seven pillars—PICERAS for short
- *Programming*, an organized plan that describes both the ingredients and the kinetics of the interactions between ingredients as the living system persists over time
- *Improvisation*, the capacity to change the programme through mutations and selection to be optimized for new environmental challenges
- *Compartmentalization*, the purpose of which is to maintain the concentrations and arrangement of the interior of each living organism and to protect it from outside
- *Energy*, life is an open energy system with some gain in entropy
- *Regenerative capacity*: The constant resynthesis of constituents of the living system subjected to wear and tear, a good example being the functioning of the heart; such a process is not perfect, and the small loss for each regeneration becomes larger, culminating in what we call *ageing*, but living systems can start over by beginning new generations
- *Adaptability*, this could arguably include improvisation; nevertheless, behavioral responses to pain, hunger, heat, or cold... obviously include another essential mechanisms of adaptation
- Seclusion for a metabolizing system with many reactions going on at the same time, is essential to prevent the chemicals of one pathway from being metabolized by the catalysts of another pathway. This property allows thousands of reactions to occur efficiently in the tiny volume of one cell, while receiving simultaneously selective signals that ensure an appropriate response to environmental changes

Two other pillars may possibly be added to the PICERAS list: The capacity to amplify gamete-like structures, and the huge security coefficient for reproduction and complexity (the billions of useless gametes...)

Still, it is impossible in 2018, to even imagine artificial life or senotherapies that don't take into account, at the least, Koshland's pillars and to restrict the senescence process to a single theory. The definition of senescence is clearly as difficult as that of life

[6, 19–23]. The SC and its secretome (the senescent-associated secretory phenotype, SASP), are central. Such a view has potentially practical applications, and has sometimes been qualified as the "geroscience hypothesis" [24, 25]. This hypothesis has its own limits and we shall try to identify them throughout the text.

The *primum movens* of ageing is the accumulation of structural alterations of chromosoms, including telomere shortening, re-expression of genes that had beneficial expression in early life and became deleterious with time, and the progressive accumulation of mutations appearing after each cell division. The overall process results in a new category of cells, the SCs, which progressively invade the whole organism. SCs are characterized by loss of the normal proliferative capacities. This deficit may have, in itself, deleterious consequences for the precursor cells of the immune system or the satellite cells of the skeletal muscle. In addition, SCs produce a number of different substances such as cytokines, inflammatory and fibrogenic factors, proteases...which generate the clinical manifestations of either physiological senescence or the chronic non-transmissible diseases, CNTD, which constitute the major problem in pathological senescence [6, 15, 17] (Fig. 1.1).

Nevertheless, it is clear that "nothing is true in biology except in the light of evolution" [26], and senescence must be placed in a broader Darwinian evolutionary

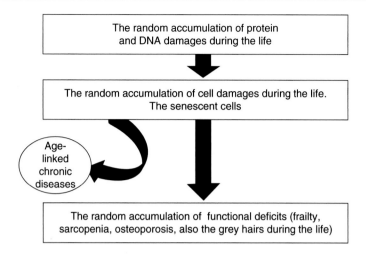

Fig. 1.1 Schematic description of the process of senescence starting with the accumulation of DNA damage and protein misfolded or incompletely destroyed. The result is an accumulation of SCs, which induce phenotypic malformations characteristic of ageing, including the age-linked non-transmissible chronic diseases

context [27, 28]. Ageing is far from being the same in every living species. Our very ancient ancestors, the nematodes, for example, got old rapidly and died from senescence within a few weeks, salmons die after reproduction, while humans live for approximately 100 years, which clearly signifies that the final net result of the accumulation of mutations during the roughly 3 billion years of evolution has increased the lifespan more than 2000-fold. For Oskar Burger [29], since 1900, the bulk of mortality has been experienced by 4 of the approximately 8000 human generations that have ever lived.

The senescent process exists in every living species, including plants [30, 31] and bacteria, and, the unsolved problem for the moment, is to know whether senescence is a universal process, being the same in every living species or, conversely, whether the process is different, even very specific, for every living phylogenetic kingdom or family (Annex A).

Nevertheless, the human being remains an exception. Since the middle of the nineteenth century, the improvement of the human mean lifespan has been due to a rapid and spectacular reduction in early infant mortality. The subsequent reduction in mortality since the beginning of the twentieth century was caused by a decline in late mortality, with a recent slowing of the process [32].

Ageing is nothing more than becoming older. From a biological or a medical point of view, ageing is a physiological process associated with a slow degradation of the diverse physiological functions of an organism, including those which are essential for life (Fig. 1.2). Ageing is said to be normal when everything is limited to a simple nonfatal degradation and qualified changes with time in anatomical, physiological, biological, and psychological structures in the absence of disease conditions, especially concerning the capacity to adapt to

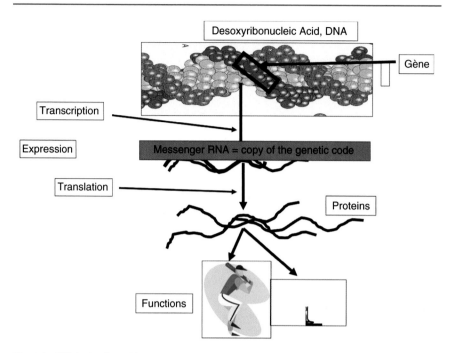

Fig. 1.2 Life is dominated by an essential paradigm, protein synthesis is not reversible

environmental changes. The senescence process is pathological when it is accompanied by one or several age-linked CNTDs. By definition, ageing is a "systemic reality" [33].

Average lifespan—or average longevity—is not fixed, the maximum lifespan is a stable characteristic for any living species [34].The maximum lifespan of the human species is around 120 years (Jeanne Calment, in France, died at 122; José Coelho de Souza, in Brazil, died at 128, although his birth date may be controversial; Emma Morano died at age 117, last year). A global analysis of the demographic data found that the present improvement of average lifespan seems to reach a plateau after the age of 100 years. Nevertheless, the maximum lifespan has remained roughly unchanged since 1990. The present progress in average lifespan probably does not affect maximum longevity and disputes concerning mortality after age 100 are likely to arise as a result of unreliable records [31]. In experimental models—yeasts, nematodes, Drosophila, mice—it is possible to enhance the maximum lifespan of the species but only using genetic manipulation [35], which hopefully will never happen in human beings.

Average life expectancy has increased regularly over the last two centuries, reaching around 80 years in 2016, and senior citizens who represented 15% of the population in 1950 will represent 35% of the world population in 2050. Such a demographic explosion will create serious organizational and financial problems [10, 36]. The mortality profile of hunter-gatherers is closer to that of wild chimpanzees than to the recent profiles of present-day human beings [29]. The main causes of death, which previously were infectious diseases, are now cancers, diabetes, CV, and neurodegenerative diseases, the CNTD [8, 9].

For a clinician, such a distinction may appear artificial, it is indeed uncommon for an old person to consult his doctor for nothing, or a single check-up, and the various small problems which are the reasons for consultation can dominate the overall clinical landscape even if they are not life-threatening. Nevertheless, these symptoms may also be the first signs of a severe fatal chronic disease. Above all, at present, we do not know whether a patient dies quietly even in the absence of any additional disease and the current problem is that, in the absence of any additional disease condition, systematic autopsies are rarely performed. The validity of national mortality registers in very old persons has been questioned [37, 38] and some authors have even shown that 30% of old people (>85 years) die from causes that would not be acceptable in younger ones. A review of autopsy findings in 200 persons older than 85 years showed no acceptable cause of death, other than complications of the ageing syndrome, in more than 30% of cases and, accordingly, it was proposed that "senescence be viewed as a disease and be accepted as a cause of death" [39].[1]

The specifics of the senescent process in the contemporary human being, i.e. the anthropogenic origin of the spectacular increase in mean lifespan, renders every wild animal (rat, mice) a model of little use in solving the problem.

1. The average lifespan of contemporary pets: dogs and cats, which are closely linked to human daily activity, is likely to increase, just like that of human beings; nevertheless, this has still not been definitely established over a large series.
2. One of the reasons why such a study is difficult is that the mortality of one of the most common pets, the dog, varies enormously according to the size (or the race) of the animal [41].
3. In addition, pets are fed with a diet which has nothing to do with their "natural" food and are frequently exposed to risks such as inactivity or passive smoking that have not been really evaluated in animals.

The notion of cellular senescence, and the role of SC and its secretome which recently emerged, allows a better understanding of the development of the senescence process and its clinical applications [15, 17, 42]. Such a view is progressively becoming predominant in biomedical literature, and instead of complexifying, it simplifies the understanding of the process and enables a better approach to daily practice [42]. This should be our guiding thread. In addition, we shall also add information on two major new scientific findings, namely the discovery by Elisabeth H Blackburn, Jack W Szostak and Carol W Greider of telomeres, and that of circadian clocks by Jeffrey Hall, Michael Rosbach and Michael Young, both recently awarded the Nobel prize (Sect. 3.3 and Annex E). Cellular senescence is, for the moment, unique in that it explains both most of the age-linked CNTD and numerous nonfatal symptoms of senescence.

---

[1] See also [5, 38, 41].

Geriatry is a medical specialty, and several books have been devoted to clinical geriatry. We can recommend two multiauthor books, one, in French, from Belmin et al. [5], the other, more recent, in English from Michel et al. [43]. These books cover the overall clinical problems, both include a chapter on the pathophysiology of senescence ("Physiologie du vieillissement" by Belmin et al. for the first; "Why do organisms age?" by Kirkwood in the second).

From a purely biological point of view, we are first inclined to describe the relationships between biological Darwinian evolution and senescence. In fact, we have chosen to start with an overview of the clinical aspects to emphasize the great complexity of the problem and the futility of any theorization. The view we select is not unique and I am fully convinced that it is still incomplete; nevertheless, this is, for the moment, the best …of the worst! The author of this book has been working for years on cardiological research and readers will not be surprised to see that the CV system represents a fairly disproportionate part of the content….nobody is perfect!

References

1. Lopez-Otin C, et al. The hallmarks of ageing. Cell. 2013;153:1194.
2. Swynghedauw B. L'homme malade de lui-même. Paris: Belin Editions; 2015.
3. Barbi E, et al. The plateau of human mortality : demography of longevity pioneers. Science. 2018;360:1459–61. (see also comments by E Dolgin, in Nature Infocus news 2018, 559, 14-15).
4. Wachter KW, et al. Evolutionary shaping of demographic schedules. PNAS. 2014;111(Suppl 3):10846–53.
5. Belmin J, et col. ed. Gériatrie. Elsevier/Masson; 2009. 835 pp.
6. Brondello JM, et al. La sénescence cellulaire. Un nouveau mythe de Janus? Méd/Sci. 2012;28:288–94.
7. Lutz W, et al. The coming acceleration of global population ageing. Nature. 2008;451:716–9.
8. GBDS, Global Burden of Disease 2016. Disease and Injury incidence and prevalence collaborators, Disease and Injury Incidence and Prevalence Collaborators. Global, regional, and national incidence, prevalence and years lived with disability for 328 diseases and injuries for 195 countries, 1990-2016: a systematic analysis for the GBDS 2016. Lancet. 2016;390:1211–59.
9. GBDS, Global Burden of Disease 2016. DALYS and HALE Collaborators. Global, regional, and national disability-adjusted life-years (DALYS) for 333 diseases and injuries and healthy life expectancy (HALE) for 195 countries and territories, 1990-2016: a systematic analysis for the GBDS 2016. Lancet. 2016;390:1260–344.
10. Ponthière G. Economie du vieillissement. Paris: La Découverte; 2017.
11. Tabuteau D. Démocratie sanitaire. Les nouveaux défits de la politique sanitaire. Paris: Odile Jacob; 2013.
12. Koshland D. The seven pillars of life. Science. 2003;295:2215.
13. Baker DJ, et al. Clearance of p16^{Ink4a}-positive cells delays ageing-associated disorders. Nature. 2011;479:232–6.
14. Bussian TJ, et al. Clearance of senescent glial cells prevents tau-dependent pathology and cognitive decline. Nature. 2018;562:578–82.
15. Childs BG, et al. Cellular senescence in ageing and age-related disease: from mechanisms to theory. Nat Med. 2015;21:1424–35.
16. Childs BG, et al. Senescent intimal foam cells are deleterious at all stages of atherosclerosis. Science. 2016;354:472–7.

17. Deursen van JM. The role of senescent cells in ageing. Nature. 2014;509:439–46.
18. Sturmlechner I, et al. Cellular senescence in renal ageing and disease. Nat Rev Nephrol. 2017;13:77–89.
19. Anderson R, et al. Mechanisms driving the ageing heart. Exp Gerontol. 2017;109:5–15. https://doi.org/10.1016/j.exger.2017.10.100.
20. Bartling B. Cellular senescence in normal and premature lung ageing. Z Gerontol Geriat. 2013;46:613–22.
21. Campisi J, et al. Ageing, cellular senescence, and cancer. Annu Rev Physiol. 2013;75:685–705.
22. Chilosi M, et al. The pathogenesis of COPD and IPF: distinct horns for the same devil? Respir Res. 2012;13:3.
23. Schmitt R, et al. Mechanisms of renal ageing. Kidney Int. 2017;92(3):569–79. https://doi.org/10.1916/j.kint.2017.02.036.
24. Khosla S, et al. Osteoporosis treatment: recent developments and ongoing challenges. Lancet Diabetes Endocrinol. 2017;5:898–907.
25. Tchkonia T, et al. Cellular senescence and the senescent phenotype: therapeutic opportunities. J Clin Invest. 2013;123:966–72.
26. Dobzhansky T. Nothing in biology makes senses except in the light of evolution. Am Biol Teach. 1973;35:125–9.
27. Frelin C, et al. Biologie de l'évolution et médecine. Paris: Lavoisier Paris; 2011.
28. Swynghedauw B, editor. Quand le gène est en conflit avec son environnement. Une introduction à la médecine Darwinienne. Bruxelles/Paris: De Boeck; 2009.
29. Burger O. Human mortality improvement in evolutionary context. PNAS. 2012;109:18210–4.
30. Thomas H. Senescence, ageing and death of the whole plant. New Phytol. 2013;197:696–711.
31. Thomas H. Senescence. 2016. www.plantsenescence.org.
32. Kirkwood TB. A systematic look at an old problem. Nature. 2008;451:644–7.
33. Lakatta EG. So! What's ageing? Is cardiovascular ageing a disease? J Mol Cell Cardiol. 2015;83:1–13.
34. Dong X, et al. Evidence for a limit to human lifespan. Nature. 2016;538:257–9. https://doi.org/10.1038/nature19793.
35. Vijg J, et al. Puzzles, promises and a cure for ageing. Nature. 2008;454:1065–71.
36. Kontis V, et al. Future life expectancy in 35 industrialized countries: projections with a Bayesian model ensemble. Lancet. 2017;389(10076):1323–35.
37. Alpérovitch, et al. Do we really know the cause of death of the very old ? Comparison between official mortality statistics and cohort study classification. Eur J Epidemiol. 2009;24:669–75.
38. Jacqmin-Gadda H, et al. 20-year prevalence projections for dementia and impact of preventive policy about risk factors. Eur J Epidemiol. 2013;28:493–502.
39. Kohn RR. Cause of death in very old people. JAMA. 1982;247:2793–7.
40. Vautel JW. Biodemography of human ageing. Nature. 2010;464:536–42.
41. Creevy KE, et al. The companion dog as a model for the longevity dividend. Cold Spring Harb Perspect Med. 2017;6(1):a026633. https://doi.org/10.1101/cshperspect.a026633.
42. Kirkland JL, et al. The clinical potential of senolytic drugs. J Am Geriatr Soc. 2017;65:2297–301.
43. Michel JP, et al., editors. Oxford text book of geriatric medicine. 3rd ed. Oxford: Oxford Univ Press; 2018.

The Emerging Medical Landscape

2

Abstract

The emerging clinical landscape is dominated by the overwhelming human responsibility and the rising incidence of non-transmissible chronic diseases including cancers, diabetes, CV, neurodegenerative (Alzheimer's, Parkinson's), respiratory and kidney diseases.

Human activity is entirely responsible for the new medical landscape that emerged half a century ago, for good and for bad. On the good side, progress in economy, medical care, food design, protection, information, and hygiene has contributed to a huge enhancement in lifespan [1]. On the bad side, human excesses are entirely responsible for climate change, sea levels, acidification, deoxygenation and desertification, pollution, and nuclear risks (see the Intergovernmental Panel on Climate Change reports, IPCC, available on Internet in several languages). The emerging landscape is strongly associated with senescence and a new epidemiological category, the age-linked chronic non-transmissible diseases, CNTD.

2.1 The Overwhelming Human Responsibility

Contemporary human activity has generated both a new medical practice and new problems in public health.[1] Some of these effects are direct consequences of climate change and the associated modifications in biodiversity (mainly microbial). Climate

---

[1] For general considerations, see [2–4]. As in many other countries, the situation of cancer in France is periodically evaluated by the *"Institut du cancer"*, INCa (see *"La situation du cancer en France"*. www.e-cancer.fr; see also Vernant JP. *Recommandations pour le troisième plan cancer.* Juillet 2013; on Internet); Jougla E. *Indicateurs de mortalité "prématurée" et "évitable".* HCSP Avril 2013. *Collection Documents;* for more societal considerations see [5–7].

© Springer Nature Switzerland AG 2019

B. Swynghedauw, *The Biology of Senescence*, Practical Issues in Geriatrics,
https://doi.org/10.1007/978-3-030-15111-9_2

change and climate warming are further biomarkers of the deleterious aspects of human activity and as such participate in the so-called "great acceleration," which includes the exponential increase in world population, pollution, urbanization, deforestation, sea levels, and acidification...[8–11] (Table 2.1).

Climate changes are clearly biomarkers (Table 2.2) of the deleterious effects of human activities [13, 14], and the classification proposed by Antony MacMichael [15] accounts for most of these remarks. For example, the reduction in agricultural production is a direct consequence of the greenhouse effect. Nevertheless, it obviously concerns a Congolese peasant more than a Berlin industrialist! The story is obviously the same for the other anthropogenic risks.

Table 2.1 The great acceleration

The social indicators
Since 1750, world population has increased exponentially from less than a billion to 6 billion, while growth in GDP has multiplied by a factor of 5 since 1950. Simultaneously, several indicators of the socioeconomic situation have also increased exponentially: the harnessing of rivers, water consumption, consumption of fertilizers, urban population, paper consumption, the number of Mac Donald's restaurants, the number of people involved in international tourism, the number of cars, the number of telephones...

The nature indicators
Simultaneously and, still, on the same exponential scale, atmospheric CO_2, N_2O and CH_4 concentrations were x 2–3
We have seen a huge increase in the number of devastating floods, drought episodes, and the intensity (more than the number) of hurricanes
The number of living species has reduced dramatically and biodiversity has suffered; microbial diversity has been modified

Table 2.2 Climate change as a biomarker. Biological and medical risks arising from climate changes. A summary

Acute risks affecting human population
The direct consequences of heatwaves (heat stroke, winter mortality) and of extreme climate change (hurricanes, floods, cold waves) and urban pollution generated by heat
The dispersion and diffusion of various pollutants and of several pathogens caused by external temperatures or by extreme climate change
Amplification of the above risks in vulnerable persons, and especially in the elderly
The diffusion of these risks due to the increasing mobility of populations and several migrations.
The direct biological effects of climate change (phenological, genetic and epigenetic effects; vernalization)

Ecological risks resulting from the climate changes
Risks mediated by changes in biophysically and ecologically based processes and systems (food yield, water flow, infectious disease vectors, intermediate host ecology)
Risks mediated by biological changes of Eucaryotes (dilution effect of vectors) or Procaryotes (Bacteria from abiotic media and microbiotes) biodiversity. New mutants due to antibiotics, herbicides, pesticides, chemicals. Immune system dysregulations

More diffuse consequences risks
Mental health problems in displaced groups, disadvantaged indigenous
Climate wars and migrations, the consequences of tension and conflicts owing to the climate change-related decline in basic resources [12], migrant flux

2.2   The Two Recent Epidemiological Transitions

What is commonly called THE epidemiological transition, qualifies a period of time, in the history of health, when, thanks to progress in the treatment of infectious transmissible diseases, the mean lifespan of the world population increased. Infant mortality collapsed and a new class of diseases emerged, the CNTD, which includes cancers, CV, diabetes, and neurodegenerative diseases. Since the end of the nineteenth century, this scenario has been more specific to the developed countries such as Europe or North America. "Epidemiological transition" was also used to qualify the fact that epidemiology no longer concerns just the infectious diseases but, in fact, every disease condition, whether transmissible or not.[2] The reduction in infant diseases was mainly a consequence of the sharp reduction in neonatal infections, which was an essential characteristic of this period.

During the last 50 years, the world medical landscape has been totally retransformed because of the considerable increase in average lifespan and the associated increased prevalence of senescent-linked problems and age-associated CNTD. Such an epidemiological transition may also be qualified as a climate epidemiological transition, although climate was more a marker than the unique cause of these manifestations. On one hand, several risks and diseases can be considered as emerging, which means that, for the moment, their incidence has significantly increased compared to the previous epidemiological situation in the same geographical space. On the other hand, the prevalence of CNTD is increasing and that of transmissible diseases has spectacularly declined [13, 18, 19].

So, the question is whether, from a general point of view, contemporary human activity does not constitute, in itself, an emerging risk and whether the changes in climate or biodiversity are not a simple biomarker of these risks. "Emergent"—by definition, requires an inventory of the health situation before and after. In practice, the response may be difficult to obtain for at least two reasons: emerging diseases are closely related to standards of living, which differ from one country or one region to another. Epidemiology is a recent science and although we have solid data concerning the present situation, data concerning the beginning of the last century were poorly documented, incomplete, and are rare. As far as the future is concerned, we also have to take into account the models selected for the climate or for the economy.

In France as in most developed countries, a state-of-the-art report is published every year. In 2017, average lifespan in France was 79.5 years for men and 85.4 years for women. Average life expectancy in good health without any severe disease increased until 2000, especially in the elderly, and the difference between men and women continues to shrink. France is characterized by an excess of mortality in men

---

[2] i.e. when Pasteur discovered bacteria and their central role, in. the mid XIXth century. Simultaneously, the discoveries of Claude Bernard, Gregor Mendel and Charles Darwin began to have medical applications [16]. See also Parascandola [17] for a historical discussion on the new concept of causation in epidemiology and its extension to every class of disease, transmissible or non transmissible.

as compared to women and by important social inequities. For the moment, globally, the two major causes of mortality are cancers (29% in 2010) and CV diseases (26%). Among the main causes of mortality, CV diseases are the main category in which mortality declined (−43% in men; mainly for ischemic cardiopathies and strokes). Cancer mortality also declined (in standardized level by age—23% in men and—12% in women). This decline was mainly due to cancers of infectious origin (eradication of *Helicobacter pylori* and gastric cancer, *Papillomavirus* and uterine cervix, virus B hepatitis and liver cancers, oro-pharynx cancers; conversely, since the rise in tritherapies, AIDS was directly involved with various types of cancers associated with this type of situation). These regressions obviously result from the beneficial consequences of human activity.

The cancer situation in France is evaluated by the *Institut National du Cancer (INCa)*. The last evaluation clearly separates cancers during childhood (1760 new cases per year, an incidence of 153/million) and in teenagers (765 new cases per year); both are rare, from cancers occurring after 65 years (365,000 new cases per year, with an incidence of 392/100,000; mean age of diagnostic 67 years). The latter belongs to the new epidemiological group of CNTD and, in France, represents the first cause of mortality. The incidence of cancers, mainly hormone dependent, increases regularly in France. A recent study showed that, after adjustments for ethnicity, education, body mass index, smoking, and age, bilateral oophorectomy before the age of 46 years was associated with a higher risk of multi-morbidity and causally linked to accelerated ageing [20]. In men, from 1980 to 2011, the incidence of cancer (in world standardized rate per 100,000 persons per year) increased from 278 to 382, and, in women, from 176 to 268, with many regional variations and, above all, many variations according to the type and location of the cancer. Progress in prevention and treatment is responsible for a significant regular decrease in global mortality from 1984–88 to 2011, the decrease being significantly more pronounced in men (−24%) than in women (−14%).

It is now possible to observe the evolution profile of nearly every type of cancer every year. It is possible to show that the recent increased incidence of cancers is observed at all ages, strongly suggesting the existence of environmental factor (s) (Fig. 2.1). These data sets can be set side by side with the well-established risk factors as tobacco smoking, alcohol, overweight, inactivity, several infectious agents, ionic radiations, various pollutants, asbestos, many endocrine disruptors, or different chemicals. For the moment it is important to prioritize these different components; it is a difficult exercise which still includes many unknowns. Nevertheless, this is, for the moment, the only possibility of detecting where we have to search for new environmental targets for preventing health damage.

2.2.1 Throughout the World

State-of-the-art reports are published every year by epidemiologists in developed countries, and also several large-scale studies covering most of the world, such as the Global Burden Diseases Study in 2015 [18, 19]. In Western countries, average

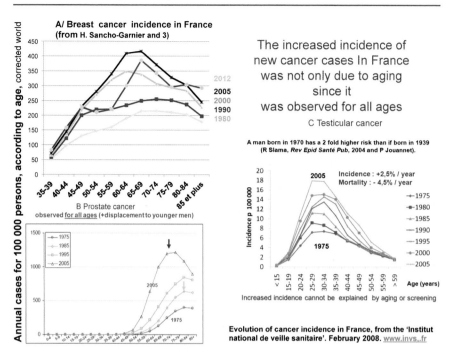

Fig. 2.1 Incidence of new cancers in France. Reproduced with permission from [21]

lifespan increased from 46 years in 1950, to 66 in 1998, and is presently around 80 years. Such an increase has mainly been caused by a reduction in CV mortality [6]. This criterion was used to establish the theoretical background to the problem in order to clarify the different regions of the world (Table 2.3). For centuries now, in our countries, the major causes of death have been infectious diseases and undernutrition. For the last 50 years, the main causes of mortality and morbidity have been CNTD, such as cancers, CV diseases, diabetes, and neurodegenerative diseases (Alzheimer, Parkinson, several types of dementias, amyotrophic lateral sclerosis). This group of diseases is also becoming the main source of economic downtimes and costs.

This epidemiological transition did not begin at the same time in every country or region, neither in every social category nor in the same city as reported, for example, by Olivier Cha (French *Académie de Médecine*, during the February 5, 2013 session), who showed that the average lifespan in persons who do not have a home address in Paris was 47.6 years, which represents 30 years less than the average lifespan of a Parisian with a personal address. In addition, the major cause of death in these persons was infectious diseases (tuberculosis is 30 times more frequent than in the average French population). The same remark was also valid for North Americans of African origin [23].

It is then possible to distinguish five different developmental stages, each of which corresponds to a specific part of the world (Table 2.3):

Table 2.3 Epidemiological models for transitions based on CV mortality

Stage of development	% of CV mortality	CV risk factors	Regional examples
Rural lifestyle, frequent hunger	5–10%	Cardiac diseases of infectious origin (Bouillaud disease)	Sub-Sahara, rural India
Recessive pandemias	10–35%	Cardiac diseases of infectious origin + arterial hypertension	China
Several neurodegenerative diseases appear	35–65%	Strokes, coronary insufficiency, obesity, diabetes	Urban India, aboriginal populations[a], former socialist countries
Neurodegenerative diseases become predominant	<50% 60/100,000 (men) in France	Strokes, coronary insufficiency in the elderly	Europe, USA
Social disturbances and regression in public health	35–55% 390/100,000 in the Russian Federation	Re-emergence of cardiac diseases of infectious origin coexisting with the previous causes + alcoholism	Russian Federation

Re-arranged from the data reported by [22]
[a]American Indians, Alaskans, native Australians

1. A stage where undernutrition and infectious diseases predominate, as in under-developed or developing countries like in sub-Saharan Africa.
2. The second is the stage where infectious and nutritional problems are starting to regress and where CV diseases are beginning to emerge, as in contemporary China.
3. Where lifespan continues to rise, CV problems become progressively predominant. This was the case for European and North American countries 50 years ago; it is now the case for urban India (current estimations for CV mortality in men from 1990 to 2020 predict a mortality of around 48% in developed countries and 127% in India).
4. In France, and most developed countries, for the moment, due to intensive preventive campaigns, CV mortality is declining.
5. Nevertheless, because of the recurrence of infectious diseases, there are countries such as in present-day Russia, in which the average lifespan is regressing.

A comparable work has been published for cancer worldwide [24]. Based on their degree of development, world regions (including Europe and USA, China, India, and sub-Saharan Africa) were subdivided into 4 groups in terms of both incidence and mortality. The most common cancers in the richest countries were by decreasing order of frequency: breast, lung, colorectal and prostate cancers, which represent about half of cancers. For unknown reasons, for the moment, colorectal cancers seem to be specific to rich countries, and cancers of infectious origin, such as liver, cervical and stomach cancers, and among these cervical cancers, are very specific to the most underdeveloped countries. In these countries, several other types of cancer are clearly more frequent, including stomach and liver cancers, followed by breast cancers, representing approximately 60% of cancers.

In 2008, the world annual incidence of cancers was 12.7%. Globally, the incidence of cancers (40%) was higher in developed countries and, in terms of world demography, predictions for the two genders for 2030 were roughly an increased incidence of cancers of around 60% (Fig. 2.1). The incidence of cancers linked to infectious diseases is reduced, but this reduction is compensated for by an increasing incidence of lung cancers (in women), of colorectal, breast and prostate cancers. We should therefore be careful when interpreting these results due to the huge heterogeneity of health registers, which differ in quality from one country to another. There is also another source of heterogeneity, which is the level of technology available for early detection of the disease; this level is highly dependent on GDP. Finally, this type of study does not account for the highly heterogeneous framework of cancers; several cancers have an infectious origin, while others depend on several toxic substances or various different pollutants.

The multiple somatic mutations, which are the origin of cancer transformation, are presently well-documented. The frequency of these mutations (expressed as the number of mutations of the exome per megabase, Mb), may vary between 0.1 and 0.2 for child cancers to nearly 10 for colorectal, stomach, and bladder cancers. The highest number of mutations (around 100 mutations/Mb, with a very high dispersion of the results—which can be attributed to exposure to highly cancerogenic products as UV rays or tobacco smoking) was reported for lung cancer and melanome. Most of these mutations were recently reported in a recent issue of the Cancer Genome Atlas. Epidemiological data have unambiguously evidenced a strong link between cancer and ageing and cancer and overweight. Another hypothesis[3] postulates that the incidence of cancer would increase because of a rise in the inflammatory risk.

The most promising approach is the analysis of the prevalence of somatic mutations. Thousands of somatic mutations have already been identified, and they already represent specific signatures. Some are common to every type of cancer, but, above all, others are linked to either ageing, or to certain agents known as being cancerogenic. The mutational hypothesis is likely to be the way that links cancer to emerging risks. It is probably the time to include in epidemiological studies the genomic data [26]. Major recent review articles concerning somatic mutations in cancers were reported by Alexandrov [27], Kandoth [28], and Lawrence [29]. The inflammatory risk and health monitoring have been suggested many times (see [30–33]). The detection of these mutations is the basis of the new approach to treating cancers.

---

[3] For example, a new mechanism has recently been proposed in a mice model which questions the production of deoxycholic acid, ADC, in some gut Bacteria induced by the feeding regime. ADC itself can induce cancer through its pro-ageing cellular effects [25]. This is a prototype of cascade mechanisms which are the origin of several dysbioses.

2.3   The Emergencies

Throughout the world, there are several major emergencies in public health; they are all the consequences of current human activity, and it is important to separate emergent risks, easy to detect, from emergent diseases which have not always been identified (Table 2.4).

2.3.1   The Two Out-Of-Control Risks: Nuclear Power and Poverty

The nuclear risk, whether it is called emergent or well-known, is obviously both 100% anthropogenic and, to a large extent, out-of-control. It has existed since Hiroshima. Physicians facing this problem are utterly at a loss for any answer. The publications on the subject are both extremely abundant and equally depressing! A recent issue of Nature ("An accident waiting to happen" Nature 2014, 509, 259) shows concerns on the place where The United States store their nuclear waste (The Waste Isolation Pilot Plan, see also page 267 of the same issue). The nuclear risk is also studied by a group of scientists—as with the IPCC for climate change—the so-called United Nations Scientific Committee on the Atomic Radiations (UNSCEAR). UNSCEAR, regularly publishes Reports, the last was on post-Tchernobyl and post-Fukushima.

These reports had reviewed the health consequences of these two events and are major references on the problem. How can we consider the nuclear risk as trivial? How can we ignore that, for the first time in the history of our planet, a few people have the capacity to eliminate all life from the planet or, at the very least, to destroy millions of people at a single touch of a button, not to mention the possibilities of a

Table 2.4 Emergent risks and diseases

For an epidemiologist, emergent risks or diseases are new risks or diseases appearing in a well-defined space or period of time. Emerging risks of human origin, like the climate risk, are global, worldwide, but their expression as a disease state may vary depending on the degree of development of the region where they occur

The emerging risks
  – Age, ageing
  – Sun's rays
  – The pollutants linked to climate change : surface ozone, fine or ultrafine particles allergens, pollens, and spores
  – Toxic risks : pesticides, endocrine disruptors
  – The new pathogenic infections
  – Agricultural yield and fishing resources
  – The "metabolic" risk
  – Flood, drought, hurricanes

The emerging diseases
  – Skin cancers
  – CNTD
  – The new infectious diseases (SRAS? Ebola, Zirka…)
  – Allergic and autoimmune diseases

terrorist placing a bomb in the chimney of a nuclear power station or the accumulation of nuclear waste or nuclear accidents linked to a nuclear power station like in Fukushima?

Poverty is the second major medical risk... obviously modifiable! The prognosis of a lung cancer occurring in a biomedical researcher is indeed much better than, that for the same disease, occurring in a person who does not have a home address or profession! Whatever the disease, the GDB, money, and education level are major risk factors and belong obviously to this category.

2.3.2 Age, the First of the Emerging Risks

The first anthropogenic emerging risk is, for the moment, ageing, which may be surprising for a new reader. The increased lifespan is neither sudden, nor recent; it has been well-documented since the beginning of the eighteenth century, with a few interruptions, due, for example, in France as in many other countries, to the last three great wars (Fig. 2.2). Nevertheless, it has obviously crossed a threshold of around 60 years.

For a living species, the first appearance of SCs is the origin of a large range of diseases which have considerably modified our medical landscape. This large group of CNTD is, in part, linked to ageing, and we now have a large group of evidence showing that SCs are directly involved in the genesis of most of the clinical manifestations of ageing.

Based on a large sample size—over 10,000 individuals annually from the 20 years of data from the Medicare Current Beneficiary Survey linked to death records through 2008—a survey from the United States concluded that disability

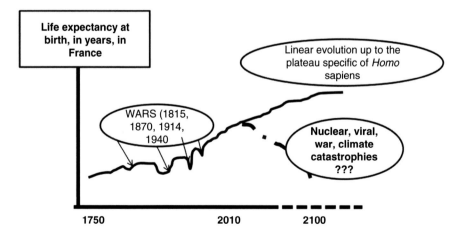

Fig. 2.2 Life expectation in France over the last two centuries. Senescence is a very specific phenomenon entirely in the hands of humans (scientists and physicians, including also crooks and mad dictators) more or less!

has been compressed into the period just before death, and that disability-free life expectancy rose and disabled life expectancy declined [34]. Definitely, we are ageing healthier.

Nevertheless, age is still the first risk. Ageing is increasing and diseases are much more frequent in the elderly, while it is, for the moment, difficult to attribute the overall origin of CNTD solely to the ageing process. CNTD are now a well-characterized epidemiological entity [5, 18, 19, 35]. The list of these diseases is fairly long and includes the majority of the CV diseases (the clinical manifestations of arterial hypertension, atherosclerosis, and atrial fibrillation), the majority of cancers (colorectal, lung, liver, and hormone cancers), diabetes, and neurodegenerative diseases (Parkinson's, dementias, including Alzheimer's disease).

How the official mortality registers match with the causes of death as it appears in the different cohorts, obviously more precise, is a real problem. A study from *INSERM* showed that the CV causes were usually underestimated, at least for the mortality of the elderly [36]. The almost explosive incidence of the neurodegenerative diseases is going to have major economic consequences [32]. In addition, a lot of data has strongly suggested that ageing is not the unique cause of these diseases, and that several environmental factors may have a favoring or an accelerating effect (Fig. 2.1). The incidence of cancer, CV disease, diabetes, and neurodegenerative disease increases regularly during lifespan, but the evolution of this incidence is not the same for the three groups of diseases over the last 20 years. The global annual incidence of cancers has increased, with big disparities according to the type of cancer; the incidence of the major neurodegenerative diseases has also increased in linear fashion in parallel with lifespan, while, in every developed country, the incidence of CV disease has declined significantly.

2.3.3 Incidence of Non-Transmissible Chronic Diseases

In France, from 1980 to 2005, the annual global incidence of *cancers* after 65 years increased significantly (from 278 to 392 cases / 100,000 in men and from 176 to 254 cases / 100,000 in women). Obviously, the question is whether the global increase in cancer incidence, which is a well-established finding, is merely a consequence of the global increase of ageing population or whether it is connected to or accelerated by one or several toxic compounds. The topic is worrisome and not entirely resolved (*Rapport Vernant* of *l'INCa* 2013 op.cit, [37]); it covers the relationships between cancer and the environment and represents, for the moment, a priority in health ecology.

The link between these emerging incidences and the new infectious, toxic, dietary incidences has been the subject of many publications. It is obviously impossible to exonerate human activity from the genesis of premature deaths (death before 65 years) and preventable deaths due to tobacco smoking, alcohol, traffic injuries, different drugs or addictions, new pollutants, new chemicals, and so on; to make such problems evident to the eyes of decision-makers still requires a lot of work!

In children less than 15 years, the incidence of cancers was not modified: 1700 new cases/year between 2000 and 2008. In men, the frequency of several cancers declined (oropharynx, larynx, esophagus, stomach, bladder, lung, Hodgkins disease, and colorectal), but the incidence of prostate, kidney, brain, testicle, thyroid cancers, and of lymphoma and myeloma increased. In women, the frequency of stomach, uterine cervix, ovarian, bladder and kidney cancers declined, while the incidence of breast, thyroid, oropharynx, larynx, esophagus, lung cancers and lymphomas, myeloma and Hodgkin disease, increased. The gender differences in incidence cannot be attributed only to hormones; they can also have cultural origins, such as the emergence use of tobacco in 50-year-old women.

The new treatments for cancers, such as radiotherapy, chemotherapy, and immunotherapy are likely to have pro-ageing effects, and a recent meta-analysis has indeed shown a significantly higher frequency of CNTD in a cohort who survived successful cancer therapy [38].

There are about more than two million cases of type 2 *diabetes* (type 2 diabetes represents about 90% of diabetes, the remaining 10% constitutes the group of type 1 diabetes that is an autoimmune disease, insulin-dependent, of young people), which represents, in France, a little more than 3% of the population, and the prevalence of the disease is increasing by 3.2% every year. The annual incidence of type 2 diabetes is about 100,000 new cases per year (about 2/1000); there are no precise data available concerning the evolution of this incidence.

In France, the prevalence of *obesity* (defined by a body mass index, BMI, >30 kg/m^2) increased from 8.5% in 1997 to 11.3% in 2003. Based on the present increase of BMI in children, it is easy to predict a rise in type 2 diabetes and its CV complications in adults in the coming years. These data lead us to think that the present reduction in incidence of the clinical manifestations of atherosclerosis could be short lived and that may not be due to insufficient therapy. Finally, we should also bear in mind that obesity is also a well-documented risk factor for cancer (above all, breast and colorectal).

The incidence of *clinical manifestation of atherosclerosis*, which is both the most acute and the easiest to quantify, myocardial infarction (the acute expression of coronary insufficiency), has declined regularly since 1980, with one exception, that of 55- to 74-year-old women, because of tobacco smoking. After 65, the reduction is—22%, in age standardized rate [39]. This reduction in incidence is accompanied by a reduction in mortality. Globally, such a reduction is due to the evolution of modifiable risk factors (tobacco, inactivity, and diet). The prognosis of coronary insufficiency is more severe in the elderly [40].

Arterial hypertension is responsible for 20–24% of CV deaths (mainly due to strokes). Prevalence correlates with age and is around 14% before 30 and 71% after 70 in men; these are, respectively, 6% and 80% in women. The relative risk of CV mortality increases with systolic pressure; the better prognostic information coming from both pressures—systolic and diastolic—more than from pulse pressure [41]. Annual incidence is around 1.34–3.04% [42]. There are no French data on the evolution of hypertension; nevertheless, there is an important world study that demonstrates a significant decline in mean systolic pressure (1 mmHg every 10 years) with major regional variations, the decrease being more pronounced in developed countries.

Heart failure is a frequent cause of excessive mortality in the elderly. A major European analysis showed that ageing is an important cause of mortality in this type of disease and is frequently associated to other comorbidities [43] (see also Sect. 6.5.5).

After 65, the incidence of *neurodegenerative diseases* increases regularly with age and their annual incidence increases every year; this group of CNTD is presently a major emerging disease. A specific study of the effects of the increase of lifespan on the incidence of dementia was performed on a cohort of 3675 subjects >65 years (mean age 75), with a follow-up of 20 years by a group of psychologists, the PaQUID cohort. Projections for 2030 have been made and conclude that at 75 the prevalence of Alzheimer's disease would be around 13% in men and 20% in women in France as in Italy. The distinction between Alzheimer's disease and the other types of dementia is not always clear in the registers and, for the moment, it is preferable to talk about the prevalence of dementia. The incidence of dementia after 85 is 38% in women and 24% in men. In France, statistical analysis of the causes of death showed a very high level of deaths due to Alzheimer's and Parkinson's diseases, which are the two most frequently occurring neurodegenerative diseases. Projections for 2030 have been made. If lifespan increases by 3.5 years in men and 2.8 years in women, which is the most likely hypothesis, we can expect an increase of dementia of around 75%. Neurodegenerative diseases are diseases of the old people; nevertheless, there are data suggesting that the links with ageing are not so simple [44–50].

2.3.4 Other Age-Linked Diseases

The incidence of several other diseases also increases with age. Ageing and the appearance of SC have variable consequences and depend on the type of organ.

The incidence of multiple *respiratory diseases* increases with age and this group of diseases is an important factor of mortality. It includes Chronic Obstructive Pulmonary Disease, COPD, and Idiopathic Pulmonary Fibrosis, IPF, and the associated forms [51–53]. Lung cancers and chronic pulmonary diseases are not the privilege of the elderly; their incidence peaks at 65 (Fig. 2.1). Nevertheless, old people frequently die from pneumonia [54]. From a functional point of view, both the respiratory capacity and the capacity of diffusion of CO diminish with ageing [55] (see Sect. 6.4).

The incidence of a number of *kidney diseases* also increases with age. Age is associated with kidneys and above all renal parenchyma atrophy (to the benefit of peritubular adipose tissue and cortical cysts). The glomerular function is affected with a progressive reduction of creatinine clearance (from 5 to 10% every 10 years after 35 years), but the tubular function is also modified with alterations of water and sodium reabsorption. The renal capacity to regenerate after stress is reduced.

Finally, renal failure is an important factor of mortality in aged persons (Rainfray in [55–57]) (see Sect. 6.4).

In 2018, age and CNTD, that are linked to ageing, shaped the new medical landscape and are the most important factors of mortality before the viral or bacterial transmissible diseases. We shall later discuss in detail the biological reasons that make age such a risk factor.

References

1. Brand S. Whole earth discipline. New York: Viking Penguin Publications; 2008. (a French version has been published in 2014 by Tristam ed Auch).
2. Aouba A, et al. L'évolution de la mortalité et des causes de décès entre 1990 et2009. Actualité et Dossier en Santé Publique. 2012;80:24–8.
3. Cambois E, et al. Ageing and health in France: an unexpected expansion of disability in mild-adulthood over recent years. Eur J Public Health Adv. 2012;23(4):1–7. https://doi.org/10.1093/eurpub/cks136.
4. Puymirat E, et al. Association of changes in clinical characteristics and management with improvement in survival among patients with ST-elevation myocardial infarction. JAMA. 2012;308:998–1006.
5. Grimaldi A, et al. Les maladies chroniques. Vers la 3e médecine. Paris: Odile Jacob; 2017.
6. Kontis V, et al. Future life expectancy in 35 industrialized countries: projections with a Bayesian model ensemble. Lancet. 2017;389(10076):1323–35.
7. Toussaint JF, et al. Croissance et renoncements : vieillir à l'épreuve du temps. Esprit Juillet. 2010;7:60–74.
8. Federau A. Pour une philosophie de l'Anthropocène. Paris: PUF Publication; 2017.
9. Hibbard KA, et al. The great acceleration. In: Costanza R, et al., editors. Sustainability or collapse? An integrated history and future of people on earth. Dalhem Worshop Report 96. Cambridge: MIT Press; 2017. p. 417–46.
10. Rockström J. A safe operating space for humanity. Nature. 2009;461:472–5.
11. Steffen W, et al. The Anthropocene: are humans now overwhelming the great forces of nature? AMJBIO J Human Environ. 2007;36:614–21.
12. Hsiang SM, et al. Civil conflicts are associated with the global climate. Nature. 2013;476: 438–41.
13. Swynghedauw B. L'homme malade de lui-même. Paris: Belin Editions; 2015.
14. Watts N, et al. The lancet countdown : tracking progress on health and climate change. Lancet. 2017;389:1151–64.
15. MacMichael A, et al. Globalization, climate change, and human health. N Engl J Med. 2013;368:1335–432013.
16. Swynghedauw B. Les racines dixneuviémistes de la révolution biologique contemporaine. Histoire Sc Med. 2006;40:141–50.
17. Parascandola M. The epidemiological transition and changing concepts of causation and causal inference. Rev Histoire Sc. 2011;64:243–62.
18. GBDS, Global Burden of Disease 2016. Disease and Injury Incidence and Prevalence Collaborators. Global, regional, and national incidence, prevalence and years lived with disability for 328 diseases and injuries for 195 countries, 1990-2016: a systematic analysis for the GBDS 2016. Lancet. 2016;390:1211–59.
19. GBDS, Global Burden of Disease 2016. DALYS and HALE Collaborators. Global, regional, and national disability-adjusted life-years (DALYS) for 333 diseases and injuries and healthy life expectancy (HALE) for 195 countries and territories, 1990-2016: a systematic analysis for the GBDS 2016. Lancet. 2016;390:1260–344.

20. Rocca WA, et al. Bilateral oophorectomy and accelerated ageing: cause or effect? J Gerontol A Biol Sci Med Sci. 2017;72:1213–7.
21. Rochefort H. Endocrine disruptors (EDs) and hormone-deendent cancers: correlation or causal relationships? C R Biol. 2017;340:439–45.
22. Yusuf S, et al. Global burden of cardiovascular diseases. Part II: variations in cardiovascular disease by specific ethnic groups and geographic regions and prevention strategies. Circulation. 2001;104:2855–64.
23. Labonté R, et al. The growing impact of globalization for health and public health practice. Annu Rev Public Health. 2011;32:263–83.
24. Bray F, et al. Global cancer transitions according to the human development index (2008-2030): a human population-based study. Lancet Oncol. 2012;13:790–801.
25. Yoshimoto S, et al. Obesity-induced gut microbial metabolite promotes liver cancer through senescence secretome. Nature. 2013;499:92–101.
26. Berger MF, et al. The emerging clinical relevance of genomics in cancer medicine. Nat. Rev Clin Oncol. 2018;15:353–65.
27. Alexandrov LB, et al. Signatures of mutational processes in human cancer. Nature. 2013;500:415–21.
28. Kandoth C, et al. Mutational landscape and significance across 12 major cancer types. Nature. 2013;502:333–9.
29. Lawrence MS, et al. Mutational heterogeneity in cancer and the search for new cancer-associated genes. Nature. 2013;499:214–8.
30. Burcelin R, et al. Immuno-microbiota cross and talk : the new paradigm of metabolic diseases. Semin Immunol. 2012;24:67–74.
31. von Hertzen L, et al. Natural immunity. Biodiversity loss and inflammatory diseases are two global megatrends that might be related. EMBO Rep. 2011;12:1089–95.
32. Pinheiro PS, et al. Cancer incidence in first generation US Hispanics: Cubans, Mexicans, PuertoRicans, and new Latinos. Cancer Epidemiol Biomark Prev. 2009;18:2162–9.
33. Rouhani P, et al. Increasing rates of melanoma among nonwhites in Florida compared with the US. Arch Dermatol. 2010;146:741–6.
34. Cutler DM, et al. Evidence for significant compression of morbidity in the elderly US population. Cambridge: Voir le site du NBER; 2013.
35. Lozano R, et al. Global and regional mortality from 235 causes of death for 20 age groups in 1990 and 2010: a systematic analysis for the global burden of disease study. Lancet. 2012;380:2095–128.
36. Alpérovitch A, et al. Do we really know the cause of death of the very old? Comparison between official mortality statistics and cohort study classification. Eur J Epidemiol. 2009;24:669–75.
37. Finkel T, et al. The common biology of cancer and ageing. Nature. 2007;448:767–74.
38. Cupit-Link MC, et al. Biology of premature ageing in survivors of cancer. ESMO Open. 2017;2:e000250.
39. Peretti C. Personnes hospitalisées pour infarctus du myocarde en France: tendances 2002–2008. BEH. 2012;4:459–65.
40. Bounhoure JP. L'infarctus du myocarde au-delà de 75 ans. In: Les effets du vieillissement sur le système CV. Paris: Frison-Roche pub; 1986.
41. Plouin PF, et al. L'hypertension artérielle du sujet âgé. Bull Acad Natle Méd. 2006;190:793–806.
42. Danaei G, et al. National, regional, and global trends in systolic blood pressure since 1980: a systematic analysis of health examination surveys and epidemiological studies with 786 country-years and 5.4 million participants. Lancet. 2011;377:568–77.
43. Komajda M, et al. The euro heart failure survey programme. A survey on the quality of care among patients with heart failure in Europe. Part II: treatment. Eur Heart J. 2003;24:464–74.
44. Baldi I, et al. Neurodegenerative diseases and exposure in the elderly. Am J Epidemiol. 2003;157:409–14.
45. Beach TG, et al. Patterns of gliosis in Alzheimer's disease and ageing cerebrum. Glia. 1989;2:420–36.

46. Collier TJ, et al. Ageing as a primary risk factor for Parkinson's disease! Evidence from studies of non-human primates. Nat Rev Neurosci. 2011;12:359–66.
47. Godet O, et al. Association of white-matter lesions with brain atrophy markers : the three-city Dijon MRI study. Cerebrovasc Dis. 2009;28:177–84.
48. Jacqmin-Gadda H, et al. 20-year prevalence projections for dementia and impact of preventive policy about risk factors. Eur J Epidemiol. 2013;28:493–502.
49. Ménard J. Rapport Pour le malade et ses proches, chercher, soigner et prendre soin. Commission sur l'Alzheimer Novembre 2007.
50. Weller RO, et al. Cerebrovascular disease is a major factor in the failure of elimination of Abeta from the ageing human brain. AA N Y Acad Sci. 2002;977:162–8.
51. Chilosi M, et al. The pathogenesis of COPD and IPF : distinct horns for the same devil? Respir Res. 2012;13:3.
52. Cottin V, et al. Pulmonary hypertension in patients with combined pulmonary fibrosis and emphysema syndrome. Eur Respir J. 2010;35:105–11.
53. Ponçot-Mongars R, et al. Syndrome emphysème-fibrose pulmonaire combinés. Revue Maladies Respiratoires. 2013;30:222–6.
54. Bartling B. Cellular senescence in normal and premature lung ageing. Z Gerontol Geriat. 2013;46:613–22.
55. Belmin J, et col. ed. Gériatrie. Elsevier/Masson; 2009. 835 pp.
56. Schmitt R, et al. Mechanisms of renal ageing. Kidney Int. 2017;92(3):569–79. https://doi.org/10.1916/j.kint.2017.02.036.
57. Sturmlechner I, et al. Cellular senescence in renal ageing and disease. Nat Rev Nephrol. 2017;13:77–89.

The Origins of Ageing

3

Abstract

Cellular senescence is the consequence of multiple factors, including genome instability, heredity, abnormalities in telomere function, proteostasis, epigenetics, and microbiota.

Ageing and the rise of senescent cells have multiple origins: genome instability, genetics and heredity, telomere attrition, abnormalities in proteostasis, epigenetics, and microbiota.

From a biological point of view, the present situation of research on ageing is similar to research on cancer. Cancerologists have proposed seven, and, recently, ten hallmarks for cancer [1, 2]. Gerontologists have proposed nine hallmarks for ageing [3, 4] (Table 3.1), which have in common three characteristics: they are all already present in normal ageing, their aggravation accelerates the senescence process, and, conversely, their attenuation improves the quality of life of the elderly. This is a

Table 3.1 The origins of ageing

The biological determinants
Genomic instability, accumulation of genetic damage (retrotransposons…)
Telomere attrition
Epigenetic alterations (retrotransposons reexpression)
Alterations in proteostasis
The homeostatic responses
Cellular senescence
Deregulated nutrition sensing
Mitochondrial dysfunction
The phenotypic response
Stem cell exhaustion
Altered intercellular connection (inflammation)

© Springer Nature Switzerland AG 2019

B. Swynghedauw, *The Biology of Senescence*, Practical Issues in Geriatrics,
https://doi.org/10.1007/978-3-030-15111-9_3

minimum, and, for example, there is certain amount of evidence that microbiota is also an important determinant of the senescent process.

"Ageing is the progressive loss of tissue and organ function over time" [5] or, to be a little more pessimistic, "a progressive loss of physical integrity, leading to impaired function and increased vulnerability to death" [3]. Nevertheless, the SC, is at the heart of the problem and since the pioneer work of Hayflick [6], the definition is the loss of the proliferative capacities of cells or the inability of a cell to divide.

The SCs are the product of genome instability and their number increases regularly with age in every organ. Cell divisions that succeed over ageing result in an accumulation of mistakes. Initially, such a phenomenon is not so important, and mainly concerns the noncoding portion of the genome, which represents nearly 95%of DNA, and, initially, does not have any significant clinical counterpart. Rapidly, before the emergence of the clinical manifestations of physiological senescence, several genomic abnormalities accumulate and, finally, the phenotype itself will be modified, either in a benign mode (grey/white hair…) or as a disease (CNTD …) (Fig. 3.1).

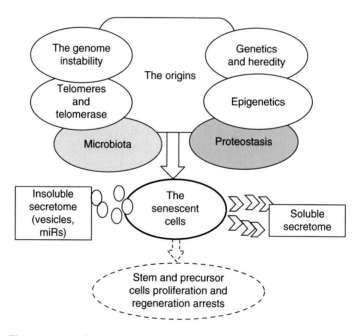

Fig. 3.1 The senescent cells are at the heart of ageing. They originate mainly from the genome instability and their progressive augmentation has clinical consequences. In addition, these cells have paracrine activity and secrete either an insoluble secretome mostly transported by vesicles, or soluble proinflammatory, fibrogenic or proteolytic factors that are, in part, responsible for the age-associated diseases

3.1 Genome Instability

Genome instability is generated by the ageing process but is also a major characteristic of cancer [7]. There are several mechanisms which allow the cells to detect and repair genome instability. The better documented of these are linked to the sirtuin family of proteins [8]. This is, for the moment, an important target in pharmacological research (see Sect 7.1). Ageing is remarkably variable from one person to another and this is likely to be a consequence of the genome instability; it has been recently attributed to natural variations in neuropeptide-mediated glia–neuron signalling [9].

The accumulation over time of DNA structural alterations is well-documented [10]. These alterations include numerous errors in replication, translocation, gain or loss of chromosomes, telomere modifications, gene cutting, modifications of the ROS (the Reactive Oxidant Species, responsible for oxidant stress). This, in turn, is aggravated both by the repair mechanisms—that have beneficial consequences and also many approximations—and by the consequences of these modifications on the spatial structure of the nucleus itself [11]. These alterations may modify the structure of either the coding or the noncoding part of the genome. Others may modify mitochondrial DNA, which has limited capacities of regeneration. The consequences of such instability are particularly important for the stem cells DNA. Repair mechanisms may also be deficient, causing accelerated ageing as in several progeroid syndromes, conversely; deficiencies in artificial reinforcement of nuclear DNA repair delay the ageing process [12].

Cell complexity not only involves the complexity of the genome, transcriptome, and epigenome, but also the spatial relationships between the chromosomal and nonchromosomal elements that make up the nucleus. This topic is at the center of the recent "4D nucleome" program [11]. This major research program aims to analyze such a spatial arrangement using biophysical technology and to understand the relationships between the 4D structure of the nucleus and the physiological properties of the cell. This is a challenge for the future and will very likely provide important new paradigms for the understanding of biology of both cancer cells and SCs. The nuclear architecture and spatial relationships of each component of the nucleus are modified. In addition, during senescence, modifications of the nuclear envelope, the lamina, are also well-documented and may cause genome instability.

Retrotransposons are mobile elements in high copy number that were active in the past and are now present as fossils in our genome. It was proposed by De Cecco [13] and Gorbunova [14] that they could result in aberrant expression or silencing of gene encoding elements controlling the immune system or homeostasis, generating genome instability during ageing. This suggests that retrotransposons may be one of the fundamental basis for genome instability of cellular senescence.

3.2   Genetics and Heredity

It is necessary to make a clear distinction between the maximum longevity of a living species and our mean lifespan, that of the twenty-first century living human being. The first is clearly genetic, transmissible, linked to Darwinian evolution (see Chap. 8). The second is slightly genetic—our lifespan may depend, a little, on our heredity, on the age of the death of your father or mother—but, above all, it depends on our environment, our diet, smoking habits, profession, and socioeconomic level.

The genetic origin of longevity is a highly complex trait and the longevity phenotype results of an intriguing evolutionary, highly population specific, and ecological mixture between environmental and genetics factors. For the moment, prominently emerged genes and DNA regions (data obtained from Genome Wide Association Studies, GWAS, Genome Wide Linkage Studies, GWLS, and whole-genome sequencing) include apolipoprotein E/TOMM40, Forkhead box O3, interleukin 6, insulin-like growth factor-1, sirtuins, chromosome 9p21 and 15q33.3. In addition, a close relationship exists between genetics of longevity and genetics of chronic age-related diseases, specially of CV diseases that are promoted by ageing. The microbiome genome is also involved and there is a need for studying the interactions between the 3 genetics components of humans, namely nuclear, mitochondrial, and microbial evidence [15].

The genetic origin of longevity for a given species at a phylogenetic level is evidence mainly for a biologist, and even more for a biologist of evolution, not for a physician. Why? Because a biologist sees both the bacteria that may live only a dozen of minutes, a nematode that lives for a few weeks, rats that live for 3 years, squirrels for 25 years, and some sharks or sequoias several 100 years. Such a gradation has necessarily a genetic origin, which is incidentally fairly complex. Such a view has been fully confirmed by experimental data and it is indeed possible to modify the maximum lifespan using genetic manipulations on multiple different genes. Undoubtedly, the longevity of a living species is plastic, but this plasticity is only visible on the time scale of Darwinian evolution [16–18].

Genetic instability is well-documented in the numerous, although rare, genetic diseases associated with accelerated ageing (Table 3.2) [19, 20]. The most frequent is the Werner's syndrome (due to a point mutation on the WRN gene on chromosome 8p12-p11.2). There are also other extremely rare diseases also associated with an accelerated senescence, the Bloom, de Cockayne, de Néstor-Guillermo, de Hutchinson-Gilford (or progeria), or de Seckel syndromes [19]. Some of these syndromes reproduce only, in part, the senescent process; others only concern the repair process.

Studies on human beings use a totally different time scale, and the data are extremely abundant. Studies based on centenarian cohorts have evidenced a modest role of heredity in lifespan (heritability 0.10-0.15); heritability is even probably lower than previously accepted and the lifespan of the progeny of centenarians was, on average, much longer than that of younger subjects. Other twin studies showed that

Table 3.2 Progeria syndromes, a summary

Names	Clinical signs	Genetics
Werner syndrome	Clinical pathology starts at 10–20 years, short stature, bilateral cataracts, early greying, hair loss, scleroderma-like skin; associated with type1 diabetes, atherosclerosis and cancers; median death 54 years	Point mutation with loss of function on ATP-dependent helicase (WRN) on chromosome 8p12-p11.2 Associated with telomere attrition and defective DNA double-strand breaks Autosomal recessive
Hutchinson-Gilford (HGPS)	Rare severe premature senescence. Alopecia, loss of joint mobility, osteolysis, lipodystrophy, scleroderma. Individuals with HGPS are not predisposed to cancer, but to have premature severe atherosclerosis; mean lifespan 13 years	Laminopathies. Dominant mutations: Aberrant splicing of LMNA (encoding the A type of nuclear Lamin A/C). The most frequent mutation is on Gly608 and causes the splicing out of 150 nucleotides, the resulting protein is progerin, defects in nuclear integrity, cell proliferation
Bloom-Torre-Machacek syndrome	Very rare, short stature, severe postnatal deficiency and skin rash after exposure to sun, increased risk for cancer and COPD; autosomal recessive; more frequent in Ashkenazi Jewish ancestry	Biallelic variants in BLM
Cockayne syndrome protein A (CSA or ERCC8) and CSB (or ERCC6)	Premature ageing with cachexia, kyphosis, retinal degeneration, short lifespan, neurodevelopmental delay and deafness	Mutation in CSA (or ERCC8) or CSB (or ERCC6)
Xeroderma pigmentosum group B complementing (XPB or ERCC3), XPD (or ERCC2) and TTDA (or GTF2H5)	Premature aging, skin cancer, excessive reactions to sun exposure, frequent microcephalies	Mutations that involved repair mechanisms of DNA. Four different types
Trichiodystrophy (TTD)	Heterogeneous group, brittle and fragile hair	Mutations in xeroderma pigmentosum group B complementing XPB (or ERCC3), XPD (or ERCC2), or TTDA (or GTF2H5) that cause deficiency in transcription-coupled repair
Néstor-Guillermo progeria syndrome	Forearm, nose and rib abnormalities, premature atherosclerosis	Autosomal recessive, mutation on BANF1
Seckel syndrome	Microcephalic primordial bird-headed dwarfism; extremely rare	One form caused by mutations on ATR

genetics may account for about a quarter of the variance of our lifespan and, for the moment, only one lifespan-linked gene polymorphism has been clearly identified, as a "gerontogene". The polymorphism is located on a gene called, APOE [21, 22]. Nevertheless, and above all, lifespan is mainly linked to environmental factors [23].

The situation is totally different for the CNTD linked to ageing. The genetic components are not the same for every type of disease. CV diseases and diabetes both have an important hereditary background; this component is still fairly important, although much more variable, in several neurodegenerative diseases.

3.3   Telomeres and Telomerase

This is becoming quite a burning issue in gerontology since the recently awarded Nobel prize [24]. The number of publications on telomeres is reaching new heights and many review articles were published on this topic [25, 26] and one more especially in the Physiological Review [27].

This discovery is an important issue for biologists. Telomeres are repetitive DNA structures located at both ends of chromosomes, that protect chromosomes against degradation, avoid interchomosomic fusions and formation of circle DNA and useless recombinations (Annex 3). These are fragile structures and cells lose a portion of their telomere after each cell division. Telomere repair is under the control of a multi-protein with enzymatic activity, polymerase. Telomerase is regulated by many cofactors that assume the security of the system, and the length of telomeres is a real biological clock, a sort of longevity certificate.

Telomere length is maintained in every cancer cell, and, in 85% of cases, this results from the overexpression of the telomerase [25, 28]. Telomerase activity is fully present in cancer cells, and is responsible for the fact that cancer cells have a constant telomere length, which is one of the hallmarks of cancer [2, 29]. Much pharmacological research was performed in order to find new senolytic therapy, based on the prolonged length of telomeres. Several research projects are still in their infancy, while the first applications are already under development; for example, favoring the survival of cells destined for cell transplantation [30].

The shortening of telomeres and the reduction of the telomerase activity are both components of the Hayflick's factors responsible for replicative senescence (Table 3.3).

Table 3.3 The causal role of telomere shortening

Telomere shortening is really a cause (or one of the causes)—the chicken, not the egg—and is likely to modify the 4D structure of the nucleus [11]. A proof of concept comes from experiments in mice [31, 32]. These authors utilized a transgenic model in which the activity of the telomerase was shut down and which presents several clinical signs of accelerated aging. Then, telomerase activity was reactivated. The final result is a regrowing of telomeres, an attenuation of DNA damage, a correction of neurodegenerescence (brain atrophy), a restoration of the activity of neuronal progenitors, and a correction of the abnormalities of the olfaction receptors

A proof of concept

3.4   Proteostasis

Proteostasis—or protein homeostasis—is an important chapter of biology and has to be precisely regulated. Proteins are complicated structures, and to be physiologically active and efficient, they require a control not only of the making of their primary structure, which is assumed, during DNA transcription, but also of their spatial arrangement and, more specifically, of their correct folding—the so-called secondary and tertiary structure (Figs. 3.2, 3.3, and 3.4) [33–37]. This is assumed by a family of proteins, the chaperones, which serve as a guide for folding, or refolding, and also by several degradation mechanisms that eliminate each useless entire or fragmented protein. The proteasomal system is responsible for the degradation of 70–80% of the intracellular proteins; it was proposed that redox homeostasis could be modulated by oxidized protein degradation by the proteasome and the circadian system [38].

Among the most prominent members of the chaperone protein family, is the group of *Heat-Shock Proteins*, HSP. The function of HSP is to assume the correct

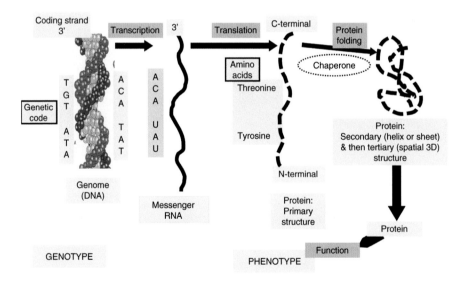

Fig. 3.2 Protein synthesis, the general consensus. DNA and its genes are the template of heredity. The primary structure of proteins results from the hereditary arrangement of the DNA nucleotides, after a first stage, the transcription of the DNA code into a messenger RNA. The second stage is the translation of the messenger RNA into an amino acids sequence, which results in the primary structure of proteins. This primary structure has to be arranged into a spatial conformation to be active. The spatial conformation includes two different processes: the secondary structure (sheet or helix) and the tertiary structure (a complicated spatial arrangement driven by chaperone proteins, which facilitate the covalent folding of other proteins). The final result is the quaternary structure, which is obtained by the associations of the different subunits. The resulting active protein is functional either as an enzyme or as a structural protein, sometimes both (such as myosin). Ribosomes and nucleus are important partners in this process and, for simplification, have been deliberately omitted from this scheme

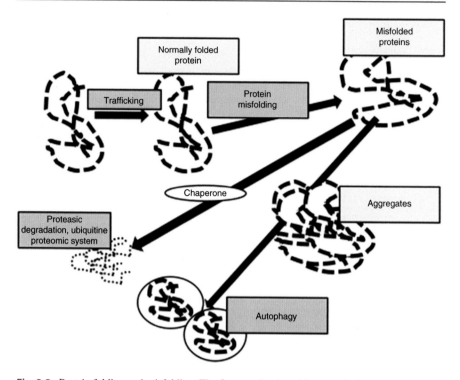

Fig. 3.3 Protein folding and misfolding. The first step begins with a protein figured in its quaternary structure. Trafficking is important to move the protein at its natural active site in the cell. Various factors, including ageing, could make a protein misfolded. The cell will have to eliminate these misfolded useless molecules either by using its proteasome, and generally by using the proteasome system linked to ubiquitin, and the presence of chaperone is crucial, or misfolded proteins aggregate and can be eliminated by autophagy. It was suggested that the proteasome activity would be modulated by the circadian clock. The latter is impaired during ageing. Misfolded aggregated proteins are known to accumulate during ageing and especially in the brain where they are likely to be a major cause of Alzheimer's disease. Notice that chaperones proteins have two functions: they allow correct folding in the making of secondary structures (Fig. 3.2); and they play a role in the degradation process (Fig. 3.4)

maturation of other proteins during formation of the spatial structure to avoid the production of abnormal aggregates with the hydrophobic groups which exist in every protein. This is a very ancient family of proteins with numerous diverse isoforms, each being specialized in a given type of repair [39]. These proteins can, by definition, be induced by stress and the stress-induced synthesis of the HSP is impaired during ageing [40]. Increasing lifespan is associated with a transgenic overexpression of chaperones, the reverse is true, and deficiency in chaperone proteins is associated with accelerated ageing [3].

The whole system in charge of the cleaning procedure, the *proteasome* complex, includes two components which are equally involved in ageing: the autophagy lysosomal system and the ubiquitin proteasome system. Misfolded proteins are normally eliminated either by the proteasome system (Fig. 3.2) or, as

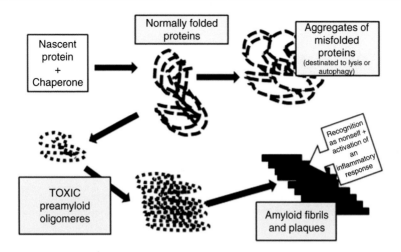

Fig. 3.4 Formation of pre-amyloid oligomeres and amyloid fibrils and plaques (in red the toxic proteins). This hypothesis is the most generally accepted, but is still a hypothesis. The accumulation of unfolded protein is linked to ageing both in the brain and in the myocardium. It may have a genetic origin or result from abnormalities in chaperone structure or concentrations

aggregates, by autophagy. Aggregates are likely to be recognized as non-self and as such, they may induce an inflammatory response [41] (Fig. 3.3). One of the pathways that regulate the first of these two systems, mTOR, can be inhibited by a chemical, rapamycin, that may have an anti-ageing and a longevity effect. Experimental studies in nematodes have shown that inhibition of the ubiquitin proteasome system extends lifespan. Inappropriate proteostasis induces an accumulation of various debris of proteins, which is finally responsible for a deficiency in physiological function. Every cell has a protection system in charge of the repair of misfoldings or of the restructuring of a normal conformation. The impairment of the elimination of these proteomic debris also participates in the general process of ageing [42].

Proteostasis abnormalities are well-documented in the central nervous system and likely to be involved in the pathophysiology of the neurodegenerative diseases. Recently, they were also discovered in other tissues and especially in the heart. The tissue is indeed rich in chaperones and in HSP (e.g., CryAB) and has both an important proteasome and an autophagic system. Mutations on CryAB cause genetic cardiomyopathy [34, 43–45].

3.5 Epigenetics

During senescence, epigenetic modifications play an important role in nuclear activity (DNA methylation, histones acetylation) [46]; epigenetic information is also, in part, hereditary [47]; DNA methylation requires the activity of an enzyme; DNA methylase, which is itself encoded by a gene. It was also proposed that epigenetic changes could be controlled by retrotransposon transcription [13]. A combination of CpG methylation sites associated to chronological ageing has been proposed as an "epigenetic clock" [48]. Epigenetics is one of the mechanisms of action of a group of molecules having either a pro-ageing or an anti-ageing effect; sirtuins that acetylate histone, and others (Polycomb), act on DNA methylation. The whole scenario is a complicated issue, very species-specific, and, for several authors, likely to be the area where future therapy should probably be developed [3]. A recent review of neural epigenetic modifications in several experimental models of neurodegenerative disease pointed out the existence of many chromatin alterations, particularly in a model of Alzheimer's disease with histone modifications that may constitute an emerging therapeutic approach [46].

Our understanding of epigenetic regulation during ageing in CV system is still fragmentary and it is still not possible to decide whether these modifications return to an embryonic state or only shift to open chromatin. Epigenetics includes changes in DNA methylation or hydroxymethylation, histone modifications, and chromatin remodeling that influence gene expression. More recently, microRNAs, long noncoding RNAS, circular RNAs, and epitranscriptome have been added to the list. The CRISPR/Cas9 technology has also been developed very recently and by more specific targeting epigenetic enzymes should facilitate the elucidation of the role of these alterations in the genesis of CV diseases [49].

3.6 Microbiota

The composition of the gut microbiota is variable, but is now a well-documented issue [50, 51]; obviously, the environment is determinant, but the genome of the person is also likely to play a role [52]. Studies on microbiota in the elderly strongly suggest the existence of an age-specific gut microbiota [49–51, 53–55]. The proposal is that the microbiota plays an important role in the regulation of metabolism and immunity and that its state may be an important determinant of certain exceptional longevity.[1]

Studies are still not sufficiently documented to enable us to affirm that, in centenarians, changes in microbiota are only linked to senescence and not just to the various diets, social customs, and ways of life that the individual experienced in his previous life. In a fairly short series, it was suggested that age may be associated with a reduced fecal abundance of phylum Actinobacteria and family Bifidobacteriaceae without any change in microbial diversity [56]. The efficiency of fecal transplantation to or from the elderly has been demonstrated, and such a therapy has been proposed as a senolytic therapy and also for the treatment of CNTD, and more specifically, type 2 diabetes and neurodegenerative diseases [51].

---

[1]A recent review article focused on healthy aging and microbiota was mainly centered on experimental approaches and did not succeeds in isolating any specific bacterial families in elderly [55].

References

1. Hanahan D, et al. Hallmarks of cancer : the next generation. Cell. 2011;144:647.
2. Hanahan D, et al. The hallmarks of cancer. Cell. 2000;100:57–70.
3. Lopez-Otin C, et al. The hallmarks of aging. Cell. 2013;153:1194.
4. Partridge L, et al. Facing up to the global challenges of ageing. Nature. 2018;561:45–56.
5. Childs BG, et al. Cellular senescence in aging and age-related disease: from mechanisms to theory. Nat Med. 2015;21:1424–35.
6. Hayflick L, et al. The serial cultivation of human diploid cell strains. Exp Cell Res. 1961;25:585–621.
7. Finkel T, et al. The common biology of cancer and ageing. Nature. 2007;448:767–74.
8. Kane AE, et al. Sirtuins and NAD+ in the development and treatment of metabolic and cardiovascular diseases. Circ Res. 2018;123:868–85.
9. Yin J-A, et al. Genetic variation in glia-neuron signaling modulates ageing rate. Nature. 2017;551:198–203.
10. Cellerino A, et al. What we learned on aging from omics studies. Semin Cell Dev Biol. 2017;70:177–89.
11. Dekker J, et al. The 4D nucleome project. Nature. 2017;549:219–26.
12. Baker DJ, et al. Increased expression of BubR1 protects against aneuploidy and cancer and extends healthy lifespan. Nat Cell Biol. 2013;15:96–102.
13. De Cecco M, et al. Genomes of replicatively senescent cells undergo global epigenetic changes leading to gene silencing and activation of transposable elements. Aging Cell. 2013;12:247–56.
14. Gorbunova V, et al. Sleeping dogs of the genome : retrotransposable elements may be agents of somatic diversity, disease and aging. Science. 2014;346:1187–8.
15. Giuliani C, et al. Genetics of human longevity within an eco-evolutionary nature-nurture framework. Circ Res. 2018;123:745–72.
16. Gems D, et al. Genetics of longevity in models organisms: debates and paradigms. Annu Rev Physiol. 2013;75:621–44.
17. Jones OR, et al. Diversity of ageing across the tree of life. Nature. 2014;505:169–73.
18. Vijg J, et al. Puzzles, promises and a cure for ageing. Nature. 2008;454:1065–71.
19. Burtner CR, et al. Progeria syndromes and ageing: what is the connexion. Nat Rev Mol Cell Biol. 2010;11:567–78.
20. Kudlow BA, et al. Werner and Hutchinson-Gilford progeria syndromes: mechanistic basis of human progeroid diseases. Nat Rev Mol Cell Biol. 2007;8:394–404.
21. Christensen K. The quest for genetic determinants of human longevity: challenges and insights. Nat Rev Genet. 2006;7:437–48.
22. Kenyon CJ. The genetics of ageing. Nature. 2010;464:504–12.
23. Wyss-Coray T. Ageing, neurodegeneration and brain rejuvenation. Nature. 2016;539:180–6.
24. Blackburn EH. Switching and signalling at the telomere. Cell. 2001;106:661–73.
25. Calado RT, Young NS. Telomere diseases. N Engl J Med. 2009;361:2353–65.
26. Cech TR. Beginning to understand the end of the chromosome. Cell. 2004;116:273–9.
27. Aubert G, et al. Telomeres and aging. Physiol Rev. 2008;88:557–79.
28. Shammas MA. Telomeres, lifestyle, cancer, and aging. Curr Opin Clin Metab Care. 2010;14(1):28–34.
29. Jesus BB, et al. Telomerase at the intersection of cancer and aging. Trends Genet. 2013;29:513–20.
30. Deng Y, Chan SS, Chang S. Telomere dysfunction and tumour suppression: the senescence connection. Nat Rev Cancer. 2008;8:450–8.
31. Hornsby PJ. Short telomeres : cause or consequence of aging ? Aging Cell. 2006;5:577–8.
32. Jaskelioff M, et al. Telomerase reactivation reverses tissue degeneration in aged telomerase-deficient mice. Nature. 2011;469:102–6.
33. Genereux JC, et al. Regulating extracellular proteostasis capacity through the unfolded protein response. Prion. 2015;9:10–21.

34. Henning RH, et al. Proteostasis in cardiac health and disease. Nat Rev Cardiol. 2017;14:637–53.
35. Kaushik S, et al. Proteostasis and aging. Nat Med. 2015;21:1406–15.
36. Labbadia J, et al. The biology of proteostasis in aging and disease. Annu Rev Biochem. 2015;84:435–64.
37. Singh SR, et al. Desmin and cardiac disease. An unfolding story. Circ Res. 2018;122:1324–6.
38. Desvergne A, et al. Circadian modulation of proteasome acitivity and accumulation of oxidized protein in human embryonic kidney HEK 23 cells and primary derma fibroblasts. Free Radic Biol Med. 2016;4:195–207.
39. Delcayre C, et al. Synthesis of stress proteins in rat myocytes 2–4 days after imposition of hemodynamic load. J Clin Invest. 1988;82:460–8.
40. Calderwood SK, et al. The shock of aging: molecular chaperones and the heat shock response in longevity and aging – a mini-review. Gerontology. 2009;55:550–8.
41. Ransohoff RM. How neuro-inflammation contributes to neuro-degeneration. Science. 2016;353:777–84.
42. Koga H, et al. Protein homeostasis and aging : the importance of exquisite quality control. Ageing Res Rev. 2011;10:205–15.
43. MacLendon PM, et al. Proteotoxicity and cardiac function. Circ Res. 2015;116:1863–82.
44. Powers ET, et al. Biological and chemical approaches to diseases of proteostasis deficiency. Annu Rev Biochem. 2009;78:959–91.
45. Willis MS, et al. Proteotoxicity and cardiac dysfunction- Alzheimer's disease of the heart? N Engl J Med. 2013;368:454–64.
46. Berson A, et al. Epigenetic regulation in neurodegenerative diseases. Trends Neurosci. 2018;41(9):587–98. https://doi.org/10.1016/j.tins.2018.05.005.
47. Margueron R, et al. Chromatin structure and the inheritance of epigénétic information. Nat Rev Genet. 2010;11:285–96.
48. Horvath S. DNA methylation age of human tissues and cell type. Genome. 2013;14:R115.
49. Zhang W, et al. Epigenetic modifications in cardiovascular aging and diseases. Circ Res. 2018;123:773–86.
50. Claesson MJ, et al. Gut microbiota composition correlates with diet and health in the elderly. Nature. 2012;488:178–84.
51. Vaiserman AM, et al. Gut microbiota: a player in aging and a target for anti-aging intervention. Ageing Res Rev. 2017;35:36–45.
52. Goodrich JK, et al. Human genetics shape gut microbiome. Cell. 2013;159:789–99.
53. Biagi E, et al. Gut microbiota and extreme longevity. Curr Biol. 2016;26:1480–5.
54. Biagi E, et al. The gut microbiota of centenarians: signatures of longevity in te gut microbiota profile. Mech Ageing Dev. 2017;165(Pt B):180–4.
55. Kim S, et al. The gut microbiota and healthy aging : a minireview. Gerontology. 2018;64(6):513–20. https://doi.org/10.1159/000490615.
56. Anand R, et al. Effect of aging on the composition of fecal microbiota in donors for FMT and its impact on clinical outcomes. Dig Dis Sci. 2017;62(4):1002–8. https://doi.org/10.1007/s10620-017-4449-6.

The Senescent Cell, SC

4

Abstract

The senescent cells and their soluble (inflammatory factors, proteolytic components) or insoluble (miRs) secretomes are at the heart of most of the clinical manifestations of senescence, including fibrosis.

Several groups of investigators have recently established a link between cellular senescence and most of the clinical manifestations of senescence. At the center of this new view, mostly based on experimental data, are the senescent cells (SCs) and their secretome. The SC is a metabolically active cell whose self-ability to repair is irreversibly reduced or suppressed because of the arrest of the cell cycle. For the hypothalamic, muscle, lung, kidney stem/progenitor cells, the reduction of these regenerative capacities has considerable clinical consequences. In addition, the SCs secretome produces in an autocrine manner several soluble or insoluble substances that accelerate or induce cancer, atherosclerosis, and neurodegenerative diseases. Fibrosis is an important, different, multifactorial, and major issue.

4.1 The Overview

Cellular senescence has been long considered as only one of the aspects of senescence, and, for most geriatricians, such a notion was the privilege of biologists and had fairly vague relationships with their clinical concerns. The concept, already very ancient, was recently enriched by several additions, the most important being from those of the van Deursen's group from the Mayo Clinic and shared by many others [1–12] who have established a consistent link between the cellular level and several of the more systemic and clinical aspects like CNTD. This work, which will be our thread, is far from being unique in supporting this hypothesis (see the legend of Fig. 4.1). In addition, it is clear that such a view is still full of several

© Springer Nature Switzerland AG 2019

B. Swynghedauw, *The Biology of Senescence*, Practical Issues in Geriatrics,

https://doi.org/10.1007/978-3-030-15111-9_4

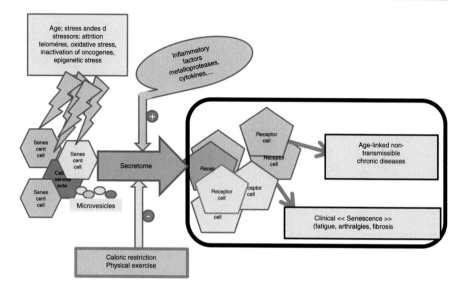

Fig. 4.1 SCs and their secretome. In this figure, SCs secrete a number of substances that form the secretome. These different factors can develop or contribute to the development of several diseases linked to ageing and also to the genesis of the fairly benign signs of clinical senescence (for example, white hair) and also of less benign manifestations of clinical senescence such as lung, kidney or cardiac fibrosis, arthritis, myopathies, sarcopenia… The composition of the secretome itself is fairly well-documented, but complex and variable from one cell SC to another, it includes, for example, several inflammatory components which participates in the so-called "inflam-ageing" and many proteases. Note in this scheme the deliberate choice of heterogeneity to describe SCs and stem cells.

uncertainties, especially in the field covered by proteostasis and in the full understanding of the pathophysiology of neurodegenerative diseases. A proof-of-concept was recently published [1] (Table 4.1).

This figure hardly summarizes the whole substance of senescence; nevertheless, it provides new views and simplifies the usual schemes of this complicated chapter of biology and pathophysiology. In addition, it provides the pharmacologist with new lines coherent with the biological view of the problem.

As such, cellular senescence comprises two different aspects.

1. The SC itself is a metabolically active cell,[1] but its self-ability to repair is irreversibly reduced or suppressed because of the arrest of the cell cycle (in the G1 phase or at the start of phase S). In addition, the cell became resistant to apoptosis and was associated with an inflammatory type.
2. The secretome, i.e. the liberation in the extracellular space by the SC of various factors (above all pro-inflammatory).

---

[1] Rodier et al. [13], defines four aspects, in part contradictory, of the SC: its capacity to both suppress and induce tumors, the senescent process itself and abnormalities in the repair processes.

Table 4.1 The role of SCs

A seminal paper from Baker et al. [1] has definitely established the validity of this conceptual framework. In a mice model of senescence, the authors were able to induce the expression of a transgene, *INK-ATTAC*, able to specifically destroy the SCs by apoptosis (defined as cells unable to divide and expressing $p16^{Ink4a}$), and only the SCs. Such transgenic manipulation increases the lifespan of both male and female mice held by different breeders. In addition, it significantly reduces the incidence of many age-related diseases of renal (as glomerulosclerosis) or cardiac origins (cardiocyte hypertrophy to compensate for an ischemic or apoptotic loss in cardiocyte; reduction in the tolerance to stress obtained by isoproterenol injection). It also diminishes the age-linked lipodystrophies. Nevertheless, protection against tumors exists but is not significant. The SCs accumulate early in adulthood and are responsible for the progressive appearance of age-linked diseases. Data suggest that the link between SCs and target cells would be the pro-inflammatory elements (such as Interleukines Il-6, Il-1a, and TNF-alpha). This is the first demonstration of a causal role of SC

Their work is indeed a real proof of concept; nevertheless, it has limitations and still only concerns rather minor clinical manifestations of the senescence process; those due to cell loss such as lipodystrophia, glomerulosclerosis, or compensatory hypertrophy of cardiocytes. In this paper, nothing was demonstrated concerning atherosclerosis, neurodegenerative diseases, or diabetes, and the results concerning cancers were not significant

This confirmation paper was recently analyzed in *Le Monde* (*Vivre plus longtemps en tuant les vieilles cellules. Le Monde Science et Planète.* February 52016)

A proof of concept

The rise in the number of SCs could result from the normal "wear and tear" of the repair mechanisms and indeed also happens after certain aggressive therapies, like chemotherapy or irradiation that may account for the senescent aspects of the tissues of patients surviving a cancer. This cell type is mainly characterized by a growth arrest;[2] nevertheless, there are both several other ways for a cell to stop divisions and many types of SC.

The scenario includes several stages:

- Firstly, cellular senescence is obviously linked to age, but it can be accelerated and even created by various stresses, oxidative, diet-induced, radioactive, SCs are products of genome instability—the term has now replaced "Hayflick factors" too limited to qualify a process that is now better deciphered. The number of SCs increases with age and SCs are not eliminated or, at least, are very slowly eliminated, because of reduced autophagy and apoptosis and also very likely because of the progressive immune decline [3, 15, 16].
- From a functional point of view, these cells are firstly characterized by an irreversible growth arrest,[3] which is associated with chromatin rearrangements and DNA damage (the DNA-Damage Response, DDR), attrition of the telomeres (and reduction in telomerase activity), and modifications of several epigenetic mechanisms (Table 4.1).

---

[2] They are also characterized by other morphological criteria that permit their identification: SCs are bigger, resistant to apoptosis, enriched in senescent-associated betagalactosidase, $p16^{Ink4a}$ and p21 [2–4, 14]. In vivo, the accumulation of this type of cell is fully documented in many experimental models and in human beings [1].

[3] Mainly due to the inactivation of the cyclin-dependent kinases that regulate the cell cycle [2].

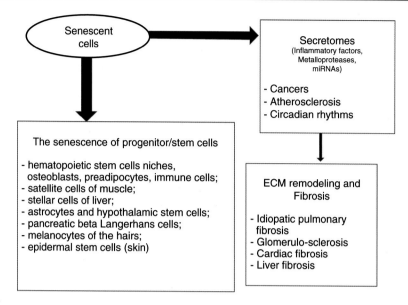

Fig. 4.2 The senescence of progenitor (or multipotent) cells and of their secretion products are responsible for numerous clinical manifestations of ageing. Extracellular matrix, ECM, remodeling, and fibrosis are apart and more complex, and may consist in either replacing fibrosis, reaction fibrosis, or fibrosis induced by a fibrotic factor from the SC secretome

- In certain cells, senescence has more specific effects. This is the case for the stem cells or for cells which possess a comparable capacity like the satellite cells of the skeletal muscle, cells of the immune system, or the chondrocytes.
- The normal secretome could be viewed as a tool, a tool utilized by SCs to communicate with each other; as such, it belongs to a paracrine system. The secretome elements are, in a large part, responsible for the fairly minor clinical manifestations of senescence (Fig. 4.2). Nevertheless, they can also induce or accelerate the diverse CNTD. A secretome is composed of soluble and insoluble elements. The latter include miRs (micro RNAs), which are transported in vesicles. Products of the destruction of a cell, for example by autophagy, are also considered as members of the secretome (see Sect. 4.3). Finally, it has also been demonstrated that the secretome of a given cell is also able to create other new cells in its proximity [6].

Since the pioneering work of Hayflick,[4] cellular senescence is defined as the irreversible arrest of cell divisions (in cell culture, subculturing is limited and is

---

[4]Hayflick was the first to show that serial cultivation of human diploid cell strains has limited capacities, indicating that cellular senescence was attained [15]. For some authors this was a direct consequence of telomere attrition. Nevertheless, it is now clear that telomeres were not the only guilty party. The history of this concept is interesting [14]. The beginning is undoubtedly the paper from Hayflick in 1961. The second step was the discovery of SC biomarkers and the work of Jeon [7] on the role of SCs in the genesis of age-linked osteoarthritis. See also, the review article of Brondello [2]. This review includes several comprehensive schemes on various aspects of this biological mechanism.

possible only 50 times); the process is clearly a protection against anarchic proliferation and cancer development. A more systemic view of the problem has been developed since this work, thanks to this new approach.

4.2   Consequences of Stem/Precursor Cell Proliferation Arrest

The cessation of the cellular proliferation is a main characteristic feature of SCs and has been observed in a number of tissues and cells. It is possible to distinguish organs, such as skin or the gastro-intestinal tract with a high regenerative capacity which use stem cells to maintain their function; organs such as lungs or liver with a slow; and organs such as the heart[5] with an ultra-slow, dormant cell turnover rate, and whose function depends on proliferation of progenitor cells. In addition, in every cases, the plasticity of resident cells is easily revealed after an injury. With age, changes in stem cells (multi-potent hematopoietic stem cells, intestinal stem cells, satellite cells of the skeletal muscle, neural stem cells, skin stem cells, germline stem cells) modify their number and function, and there are also stem cells that are resistant to ageing. The position of these cells which are at the base of cellular lineages renders their dysfunction potentially more impactful than that of other cells [18, 19] and obviously explains many clinical data (Fig. 4.2, Table 4.2) (see below Sect. 5.3).

Table 4.2 The clinical consequences of the apparition of senescent cells

– *Hypothalamic stem cells, microglia, and astrocytes; the phosphorylation of tau protéins* (neurodegenerative diseases)
– *Skeletal muscle satellite cells* (sarcopenia)
– *Keratinocytes in the skin* (loss of elasticity)
– *Osteoclasts* (osteoporosis) *and chondrocytes* (osteoarthritis)
– *Adipocytes and preadipocytes* (obesity and lipodystrophies)
– *Kidney: tubular atrophy and reduction in the number of nephrons* (renal failure)
– *Pancreatic beta Langerhans cells* (diabetes)
– *Lung: epithelial and alveolar cells, fibroblasts* (COPD, IPF)
– *Liver: stellar cells* (cirrhosis)
– *Heart: reduction in the number of myocytes and vascular epithelium* (reduced function, heart failure)
– *Hair melanocytes and hair color*
– *Hematopoiesis* (anemia) *and immune cells* (immunosenescence, also bone and adipose tissue)

---

[5] Recently, Ronaldson-Bouchard [17] have reported an interesting new model for generating cardiac tissue. In this model, they utilized early-stage human-induced pluripotent stem cells-derived cardiocytes to stimulate the formation of cardiac tissue. The cardiac stem cell system is present, although dormant.

1. Hematopoietic stem cells reside in the bone marrow and the number of active stem cells declines with age, with a tendency to differentiate toward the myeloid lineage at the expense of the lymphoid lineage. The functional deterioration of the immune system with age, also called immunosenescence, has been demonstrated on both on innate and adaptive systems. Old stem cells transferred to young hosts retain their aged phenotype, suggesting that ageing in this category of cells is driven by cell-intrinsic mechanisms [18, 20].

2. The stem cells of the skeletal muscle consist of a small population of cells called satellite cells in charge of the renewal and repair of these cells, particularly after exercising or injury; ageing is associated with a reduction in the number of these satellite cells. Aged satellite cells exhibit a skewed differentiation potential and tend to differentiate into fibroblast and to create muscle fibrosis. The same is true for the osteoblasts and osteopenia is frequently associated with sarcopenia [21].

3. The senescent chondrocytes secretome is enriched in proteases and inflammatory factors and, as such, has a high potential for destroying the extracellular matrix, ECM, and it is now fairly well-established that the senescent phenotype may generate osteoarthritis and the synovial hypertrophy, which is associated with this disease condition.

4. Adipose tissue, which is, usually, the largest organ in humans, is strongly modified by ageing. Preadipocytes, which are fat cell progenitors close to macrophages, and comprising 15% of cells in fat, dedifferentiate and progressively switch to SC (as indicated by the presence of specific biomarkers, like beta galactosidase) and acquire a secretome, which is increasingly enriched in inflammatory components. With ageing, there is a decline in preadipocyte replication, decreased adipogenesis associated with a reduction in adipogenic transcription factors, and an increase in pro-inflammatory elements. With ageing, this tissue, and more specifically preadipocytes, lose their ability to store the toxic fatty acids, activate the immune response, and become a major source of inflammatory factors [22].

5. The pancreatic Langerhans beta cells have a fairly limited replication potential, and in nutrient-induced diabetic mice fed with a diet enriched in lipids, pancreatic senescence aggravated the diabetic markers [23].

6. With ageing, neural stem cells decrease in number; nevertheless, there are data that strongly suggest that extrinsic factors were at play in the neuronal ageing process and recently, two seminal papers [24, 25] have unambiguously demonstrated in mice that the adult neural stem/progenitor cells located in the mediobasal region of the hypothalamus were a major determinant in the senescence process. It was demonstrated in experimental models that the SCs also plays a causal role in the hyperphosphorylation of tau proteins [26] (see Sect. 6.2).

7. The regenerative capacity of the kidney, like for other tissues, after a traumatism or a transplantation, is reduced with age [11, 27]. Liver aggressions induce the

proliferation of stellar cells which originate from liver fibrosis and steatosis, leading finally to cirrhosis. The accumulation of SCs in the liver generates non-alcoholic steatosis and the number of SCs in the liver correlates with the degree of steatosis. Conversely, the transgenic or therapeutic reduction in SCs number attenuates the degree of steatosis [28].

8. The gut epithelium of mammalians has, under normal conditions, an extremely rapid turnover and contains two interconvertible populations of stem cells; a proliferative one in the base of the crypt and another more quiescent one above the crypt. Some data suggest that the change in stem cells in an aged intestine may contribute to the increase in the incidence of colorectal cancer. Data in human beings are fairly rare and most of our knowledge comes from the study of Drosophila, a living species quite removed from clinical concerns!

9. The decline in fertility with ageing is undoubtedly a crucial point during the history of any living species. In males, the germline is maintained by the spermatogonial stem cells and declines with ageing. In females, the germline stem cells are called oogonial stem cells.

4.3   The SC Secretome

Secretome components are highly variable from one cell to another; they are either soluble or insoluble inside microvesicles made from the external membrane of the cell, the exosomes [12, 29]. The secretome is becoming an important potential pharmacological target in geriatric [1].

A secretome is the product of either paracrine secretory activity or of a simple autophagic process. It requires the pre-existence of genomic or epigenetic damage in the SCs, the "senescent-associated secretory phenotype", SASP. The autophagic

Table 4.3   miRs in ageing and age-related CNTD

Aged persons without any associated diseases	Increased inflammation-associated miRs (miR-146a)
Alzheimer	Increased miRs associated with inflammation (miR-9, -146a, -125b, -155) and miR31
Rheumatoid arthritis (synovial fluid)	Increased miR-155
Cancers	Inflamma-miRs (above all miR-146a and miR-21) are modulators of cancer development
Type 2 diabetes	miR-21 and miR-126 are reduced, some were proposed as serum markers
Clinical manifestations of atherosclerosis	Several miRs are secreted by endothelial cells and play a role either as a trigger or as a bio-protector: mir-143 and miR-145 prevents the dedifferentiation of vascular cells; miR-126 activates the production of pro-inflammatory factors

process is also called "communicome". The secretome contains several metalloproteases, the MMPs, that regulate the composition of the extracellular matrix, ECM, several pro-inflammatory factors, such as interleukins IL-6, IL-8, TNF-1alpha, several activators of cellular proliferation such as the growth-regulated oncogenes, GROs, and growth factors and miRs (miR21, for example is at the intersection point between ageing /inflammation/CNTD) [30] (Table 4.3). Others have suggested other elements like myokines (myostatin and follistatin, its inhibitor, for sarcopenia, and the brain-derived neurotrophic factor, BDNF, and interleukin, IL-6 for lipodystrophies and age-linked obesity [31, 32].[6] (Table 4.1 and Annexes C and D).

The blood or cerebrospinal fluid contents in secretome products are also well-documented by several proteomic studies [31]. Age-linked secretome composition is fairly well-documented; nevertheless, its composition depends on three variables, age, time and cellular type, and, at present, such an approach has not resulted in any practical clinical applications and the link with one of CNTD has not been unequivocally demonstrated [33].

4.4   Fibrosis

Age is associated with tissular fibrosis, which is a different problem. Some years ago, it was common to distinguish replacement fibrosis: fibrosis wherein a portion of the tissue lost is replaced after ischemia like the scar after a myocardial infarction, apoptosis or a traumatism, and reactive fibrosis that happens after an inflammation process [34]. It is difficult to qualify fibrosis during senescence, because it is usually a mixture of the two, and a third type of fibrosis has to be added, fibrosis due to the senescent process itself, which is under the control of the fibrogenic factors present in the SC secretome [19, 34–38]. To further complicate the problem, there are also data showing that with age, several groups of stem cells, like the satellite cells of the skeletal muscle, may dedifferentiate toward a fibrotic lineage. During ageing, several organs, at the least, may be affected by fibrosis, including the lungs, liver, heart and kidneys. Lens has been proposed as an avascular model to study fibrosis [19, 34–39] (Table 4.4).

---

[6]An extensive study quantified more than a thousand different blood proteins in two large female groups (age range 39–83 years) based on the high throughput SOMA proteomics approach (the-SOMAmer-based capture array) and identified 11 proteins with a very low heritability and whose levels were significantly increased with age. The strongest association was with chordin protein like 1 (an antagonist of the bone morphogenetic protein 4, also involved in angiogenesis and stem cell development, strongly linked to birth weight) and pleiotrophin (a multifunctional growth factor known as a CV marker). Other, s linked to ageing were identified, like the insulin-like growth factor, IGFBP-6, and MMP-12. Nevertheless, this paper emphasizes that care should be taken when using some of these proteins as markers of ageing because some of these high levels of proteins were also correlated with lower predicted CV risks and birth-weight [31].

Table 4.4 Fibrosis is not unique, a profusion of mechanisms and targets

Fibrosis qualifies an increased concentration of tissue collagen. The collagen gene is a particular gene composed of repetitive sequences and its synthesis is a complicated phenomenon, largely not regulated on the transcriptional level as shown in our laboratory
During development, collagen synthesis normally increases in proportion to the increased tissue mass with an unchanged concentration; this is not fibrosis. Fibrosis, a wounding response, proceeds in several steps, including activation of effector cells, elaboration of the extracellular matrix, and a dynamic deposition of ECM [34]
Collagen is an extremely stiff protein, which ultimately promotes end organ failure in heart, kidneys, lungs, lens, liver…
Fibrosis can be replacement fibrosis, reactive fibrosis, or a response to fibrogenic factors, such as those present in the SCs secretome
The proliferation of myofibroblasts and fibroblasts are key elements in every organ, together with TGF-beta cascade, which is a potent activator of the synthesis of extracellular matrix components. Epigenetic regulation is important in fibrogenesis.
Fibrosis can be reversed for example by the activation of the group of metallo-proteases, but also by several therapies, including anti-aldosterone, or angiotensin-converting enzyme inhibitors

References

1. Baker DJ, et al. Naturally occurring p16^{Ink4a}-positive cells shorten healthy lifespan. Nature. 2016;530:184–9.
2. Brondello JM, et al. La sénescence cellulaire. Un nouveau mythe de Janus. Méd/Sci. 2012;28:288–94.
3. Campisi J, et al. Ageing, cellular senescence, and cancer. Annu Rev Physiol. 2013;75:685–705.
4. Childs BG, et al. Cellular senescence in ageing and age-related disease: from mechanisms to theory. Nat Med. 2015;21:1424–35.
5. Chung HY, et al. Molecular inflammation : underpinnings of ageing and age-related diseases. Ageing Res Rev. 2009;8:18–30.
6. Deursen van JM. The role of senescent cells in ageing. Nature. 2014;509:439–46.
7. Jeon OH, et al. Local clearance of senescent cells attenuates the development of post-traumatic osteoarthritis and creates a pro-regenerative environment. Nat Med. 2017;23:775–82.
8. Jurk D, et al. Chronic inflammation induces telomere dysfunction and accelerates ageing in mice. Nature Commun. 2014;5:4172. https://doi.org/10.1038/ncomms5172.
9. Kirkland JL, et al. Cellular senescence: a translational perspective. EBioMedicine. 2017;21:21–8.
10. Malaquin N. Keeping the senescence secretome under control : molecular reins on the senescence-associated secretory phenotype. Exp Gerontol. 2016;82:39–49.
11. Sturmlechner I, et al. Cellular senescence in renal ageing and disease. Nat Rev Nephrol. 2017;13:77–89.
12. Weilner S, et al. Secretion of microvesicular miRNAs in cellular and organismal ageing and age-related diseases. Exp Gerontol. 2013;48:626–33.
13. Rodier F, et al. Four faces of cellular senescence. J Cell Biol. 2011;192:547–56.
14. Childs BG, et al. Senescent cells: an emerging target for diseases of ageing. Nat Rev Drug Discov. 2017;16:718–35.
15. Hayflick L, et al. The serial cultivation of human diploid cell strains. Exp Cell Res. 1961;25:585–621.
16. Jeyapalan JC, et al. Accumulation of senescent cells in mitotic tissues of ageing primates. Mech Ageing Dev. 2007;128:36–44.

17. Ronaldson-Bouchards K, et al. Advanced maturation of human cardiac tissue grown from pluripotent stem cells. Nature. 2018;556:239–43.
18. Schultz MB, et al. When stem cells grow old: phenotypes and mechanisms of stem cells ageing. Development. 2016;143:3–14.
19. Wells JM, et al. Diverse mechanisms for endogenous regeneration and repair in mammalian organs. Nature. 2018;557:322–8.
20. Panda A, et al. Human innate immunosenescence: causes and consequences for immunity in old age. Trends Immunol. 2009;30:325–33.
21. Hirschfeld HP, et al. Osteosarcopenia: where bone, muscle and fat collide. Osteoporos Int. 2017;28(10):2781–90. https://doi.org/10.1007/s00198-017-4151-8.
22. Tchkonia T, et al. Cellular senescence and the senescent phenotype: therapeutic opportunities. J Clin Invest. 2013;123:966–72.
23. Sone H, et al. Pancreatic beat cell senescence contributes to the pathogenesis of type 2 diabetes in high-fat diet-induced diabetic mice. Diabetologia. 2005;48:58–67.
24. Zhang G, et al. Hypothalamic programming of systemic ageing involving IKK-beta, $NF_{-kappa}B$ and GnRH. Nature. 2013;497:211–6.
25. Zhang Y, et al. Hypothalamic stem cells control ageing speed partly through exosomal miR-NAs. Nature. 2017;548:52–7.
26. Bussian TJ, et al. Clearance of senescent glial cells prevents tau-dependent pathology and cognitive decline. Nature. 2018;562:578–82.
27. Bartling B. Cellular senescence in normal and premature lung ageing. Z Gerontol Geriat. 2013;46:613–22.
28. Ogrodnik M, et al. Cellular senescence drives age-dependent hepatic steatosis. Nat Commun. 2017;8:15691. https://doi.org/10.1038/ncomms15691.
29. Waldenström A, et al. Role of the exosomes in myocardial remodeling. Circ Res. 2014;114:315–24.
30. Olivieri F, et al. Circulating inflamma-miR in ageing and age-related diseases. Front Genet. 2013;4:1–9.
31. Menni C, et al. Circulating proteomic signatures of chronological ages. J Gerontol A Biol. 2015;70:809–16.
32. Pedersen BK, et al. Muscles, exercise and obesity : skeletal muscle as a secretory organ. Nat Rev Endocrinol. 2012;8:457–65.
33. Naylor RM, et al. Senescent cells : a novel therapeutic target for ageing and age-related diseases. Clin Pharmacol Ther. 2013;93:105–16.
34. Weber KT. Wound healing in cardiovascular disease. Armonk: Futura Publishing Company; 1995.
35. Hashimoto M, et al. Elimination of p19ARF-expressing cells enhances pulmonary function in mice. JCI Insight. 2016;1:e87732.
36. Rockey DC, et al. Fibrosis – A common pathway to injury and failure. N Engl J Med. 2015;372:1138–49.
37. Schafer MJ, et al. Cellular senescence mediates fibrotic pulmonary disease. Nat Commun. 2017;8:1–11.
38. Weber KT, et al. Myofibroblasts-mediated mechanisms of pathological remodeling of the heart. Nat Rev Cardiol. 2013;10:15–26.
39. Elred JA, et al. The lense as a model for fibrotic disease. Philos Trans R Soc Lond B Biol Sci. 2011;366:1301–19.

The Nonfatal Clinical Manifestations of Ageing

5

Abstract

Most of the nonfatal clinical manifestations of senescence—including grey hairs, adipose tissue dysfunctioning, osteoporosis, osteoarthritis, sarcopenia and also the frailty syndrome, immunosenescence, and changes in biological rhythms (mostly circadians)—are linked to the secretome of senescent cells.

It is possible to separate the nonfatal manifestations from the fatal ones, the latter, roughly speaking, covering CNTD. Ageing is associated with various clinical traits such as grey hair, impaired wound healing, or osteoporosis, osteoarthritis and sarcopenia, or the frailty syndrome and disorders in the immune system. There is an established link between modifications of the circadian rhythms and SCs, which has considerable consequences for sleep and thermoregulation, and several other pathways. There is a profusion of metrics of ageing; nevertheless, a study of the hierarchical domains in ageing is still lacking [1].

We realize that, obviously, such a distinction could be considered as artificial for any clinician who is faced every day with the complicated history of each of his aged patients [2] (Table 5.1).

5.1 Hair, Skin, Adipose Tissue

Hair becomes rare and grey when hair follicles that sustain both hair growth and pigment-producing melanocytes cease functioning. This form of senescence, like every form of ageing, can be accelerated by environmental phenomena such as stress. Stress-induced tonsure such as scalp separation, for example, is well-known to every hair-dresser!

Ageing reduces the self-renewing capacity of the *skin* epiderma and aged skin resembles skin chronically exposed to solar UV (photoageing). Skin has two main

© Springer Nature Switzerland AG 2019

B. Swynghedauw, *The Biology of Senescence*, Practical Issues in Geriatrics,

https://doi.org/10.1007/978-3-030-15111-9_5

Table 5.1 The clinical manifestations of senescence

Skin, hair, adipose tissue
- Hair greying and skin wrinkling
- Impaired wound healing
- Lipodystrophies

Bones and joints
- Osteoporosis
- Osteoarthritis
- Sarcopenia
- Osteosarcopenia

General conditions
- Frailty
- Immunosenescence
- Colon diverticulosis
- Reduced physiological complexity and progressive impairment of adaptive responses to the numerous stressors of life (respiratory dynamics, heart beats, postural control, locomotor system, manual force production, and brain networks) (see Annex B).

Biological rhythms
- Changes in circadian rhythms
- Sleep disorders
- Thermoregulation

The five senses
- Presbyacusia
- Presbyopia
- Cataract
- Anorexia and impairments in smell and taste

The universal ageing trait

physiological properties: it is a barrier against any intrusion and a thermoregulator; and, as such, skin alterations may have important consequences for aged persons. When keratinocytes stop proliferating, the result is a thinning of the epiderma and delayed wound healing [3]; nevertheless, there are also data suggesting that the secretome of SCs would stimulate tissue repair and help to resolve fibrosis in the wound [4]. Proteases from the secretome also play a role in the loss of skin elasticity and the gradual fragmentation of the dermal collagenous extracellular matrix.

Adipose tissue has two vital physiological functions: it stores energy and maintains thermoregulation. It also produces several hormones, such as angiotensin II, leptin, adiponectin, IL-6 and IGF-1, and activates other hormones such as glucocorticoids and the sex steroid. This tissue also has two unusual properties: it is rarely infected by bacteria or viruses and metastases are very uncommon. These properties are likely related to the innate and adaptive immune elements present in this tissue. In old persons, fat is redistributed from subcutaneous to intra-abdominal visceral depots with various ectopic depositions. *Obesity* and *lipodystrophies* are linked to ageing for many reasons, including inactivity and solitude. During ageing, lipolysis is reduced by 50% and this deficit has been attributed to a reduction in the adipose tissue lipase activity; at present, there is no explanation for this phenomenon [5]. Lipase deficiency may be responsible for the aged-linked changes in thermoregulation, the reduction in physical activity, and the redistribution of fat. Recently, Camell et al. [6] evidenced a link between the catecholamine-induced diminution of lipolysis and obesity.

From certain aspects, the adipose tissue of obese persons could be considered as an accelerated form of aged adipose tissue ([7] proposed an interesting model based on this concept). The crucial role of the adipose tissue in senescence is becoming more and more evident. Pre-adipocytes, which are the progenitors of the adipose cells, and other mesenchymatous cells, dedifferentiate with ageing, and when they become SCs, acquire major inflammatory properties.

5.2   Bones, Muscles, and Joints

Osteoporosis and its deleterious complications are a frequent complication of ageing (in 2000, about nine million osteoporotic patients were identified worldwide; osteoporosis is frequently associated with multiple comorbidities). Osteoclasts are mechanosensors adapted to the mechanical environment and emit signals that regulate the osteoblast and osteoclast number, and bone frailty is linked to both a reduced osteocytes number and to their own senescence, i.e. the loss of their replicative ability. Senescent osteocytes have reduced mechanoreceptive properties. Several genetic polymorphisms and endocrine dysfunctioning are also linked to osteoporosis. This is a field where the therapeutic applications are the most promising. Bone marrow mesenchymal stem/stromal cells may differentiate into osteogenic, adipogenic, myogenic, and chondrogenic lineages to support the muscle and bone development and tissue homeostasis, and with ageing, osteogenesis and bone formation decrease while marrow adipogenesis increases [8–10].

The loss of skeletal muscle mass in the elderly, whether it is included in the frailty syndrome or not, is a major clinical problem for any geriatrician. *Sarcopenia* was the term, first coined by Rosenberg in 1989, which includes both the loss of muscle mass and reduced muscle strength. These are dissociated factors. In ageing, the capacity of the muscle progenitor cells, the satellite cells, to regenerate after healing is reduced. The satellite cells are modified by epigenetic mechanisms: alterations of the DNA methylation and histone acetylation that modify Hoxa expression. The Hoxa de-repression has been proposed as a therapy for sarcopenia [11–17].

In contrast to type I muscle fiber, type II skeletal muscle fiber size was substantially smaller with ageing and this was accompanied by an age-related reduction in type II muscle fiber satellite cell content. Twelve weeks of resistance-type exercise training increased type II muscle fiber size and satellite cell content, strongly suggesting that training may represent an effective strategy to reverse muscle atrophy. Sarcopenia is preceded by a loss of the motor units, without any compensatory hypertrophy of the remaining units and there is evidence of an age-related decline in motor unit recruitment and in motor unit discharge rate. In addition, sarcopenic elderly subjects fail to expand the motor unit size to compensate for declining motor unit numbers. A meta-analysis, based on 772 references, showed a significant higher rate of mortality among sarcopenic subjects, and an associated functional decline, with a higher rate of falls and hospitalizations [11, 14, 18–20].

Premature cartilage senescence is the basis of *osteoarthritis* and is one of the nonfatal diseases, the most familiar to every geriatrician. Osteoarthritis is associated with multiple mechanical stresses and the critical role of senescent chondrocytes is well-documented. Their secretome is rich in proteases and inflammatory factors that degrade the cartilages and the senescent phenotype of chondrocytes is strongly associated with osteoarthritis and participates in the associated synovial hypertrophy. Senescent chondrocytes have short telomeres, unstable genomes, and several epigenetics defects characteristic of SCs. After a traumatism, the experimental removal of SCs from joints suppresses the clinical manifestations of osteoarthritis [21–24].

5.3 General Conditions, Frailty Syndrome, Fluid Balance, Immune System

Frailty is the main component of a physiological syndrome that affects the functions dependent on energetics and the speed of performance or mobility. A biologically-based theory regarding the phenotype of *frailty* was developed by Linda Fried [25], which definitively established a standardized clinical definition of frailty, and the *frailty syndrome*, in community-dwelling older adults. Frailty is associated with disability and comorbidity, although frailty is not synonymous with comorbidity or disability. Frailty is present when the following criteria are associated: unintentional weight loss and sarcopenia, self-reported exhaustion, weakness, slow walking speed, and low physical activity. Frailty is linked to socioeconomic status and is associated with a number of major chronic diseases. Fat infiltration may also be prevalent; osteoporosis, and osteosarcopenia are frequently included in the definition of the syndrome: "osteosarcopenia: where bone, muscle, and fat collide" [18]. A position paper from the French society of geriatrics and gerontology defined frailty in the elderly as a reduction of the adaptation capacity to stress, which must be predictive of functional decline and adverse outcomes [26].

Fluid balance is usually normal in old persons, but the response to acute situations, such as dehydration, is impaired. Reduced thirst in response to dehydration is a well-documented phenomenon in elderly humans and animal models of ageing, it is associated with a reduced sodium appetite and several alterations in endocrine systems involved in maintaining electrolyte homeostasis. The activity of the renin angiotensin aldosterone is reduced, with a lower plasma renin, and a substantial enhancement of the plasma atrial and brain-natriuretic and arginine vasopressin [27].

Both the production of the progenitor cells of the *immune adaptive system* and *hematopoiesis* are reduced with ageing. In addition, there are qualitative changes in the innate immune system, which becomes less efficient in its capacity to couple with the adaptive system, with a reduction in the number of receptors [28, 29]. Nevertheless, immunosenescence is a more complex issue and also includes a rise in the plasma concentrations of several inflammatory factors as a constitutive pro-inflammatory environment, the so-called "inflammaging" (see Sect. 8.2). There is evidence that there is an age-related increase in inflammatory cytokines of the secretome and that this elevation reflects an increased output from both mono-cytes and stromal cells, like the fibroblasts. Then, immunosenescence appears to be more a dysregulation of the immune system than an exclusive impaired func-tioning [29, 30].

The two components of *the immune system*—the adaptive system and the innate system—interplay in the genesis of the immune response and both are modified with ageing. One of the consequences is a reduction of the capacity to respond to a bacterial or a viral infection with ageing. Both terminally differentiated T cells and B cells are less efficient. For example, in a recent study, clinical evidence was pro-vided for an age-related defect in the Toll-like Receptor, TLR, in human macro-phages in the context of a viral infection with a disproportionately high morbimortality in the elderly.

New blood cells are produced from stem cells of *the hematopoietic system* in the bone marrow, which have a very high turnover rate. With ageing, their regenerative potential is reduced and among the consequences of this impaired tissue homeosta-sis is a moderate *anemia*, frequently observed in the elderly, and an increased inci-dence of myeloid proliferative diseases. Hematopoietic stem cells are located along the bone surface and form two niches: the endosteal, which also includes osteo-blasts; and vascular niches [30, 31]. The study of endothelial development has been intertwined with hematopoiesis for a long time ever since a bipotential cell, the hemangioblast, was noted as producing both endothelial and hematopoietic cells, and clearly, the two systems have a direct lineage end origin, the hemogenic endo-thelium [32].

> The immune system present in the vast mucosa of the *gut* is also affected by immunosenes-cence, which reduces adaptability and affects digestion, the relations with microbiota and will, finally, result in an increased morbidity in elderly [33].

There is a well-documented age-dependent augmentation of both the prevalence of thromboembolic events [34, 35], mainly caused by the frequency of the clinical manifestations of atherosclerosis and bleeding complications during antithrombotic therapy [36], mainly linked to chronic kidney diseases [37]. So far, several modifi-cations of the *coagulation* factors have been reported in aged persons, including an increased fibrinogen concentration, factor X, and also an augmentation of most of the coagulation proteins [38, 39]. Globally, there is a shift of the hemostatic balance toward an increased clotting time and decreased fibrinolysis [37, 38] (Fig. 5.1). The augmentation of plasma fibrinogen has been confirmed in a proteomic study on a population of 240 healthy individuals, 22–93 years old, that has identified 197 pro-teins positively and 20 proteins negatively associated with age using the SOMAscan technology. Using the GO term cluster targeted the authors were able to identify several functional groups. Among them, the blood coagulation cluster increases with ageing together with fibronectin, both being related to the inflammatory state. Interestingly, this proteomic approach also provides data showing an enrichment of

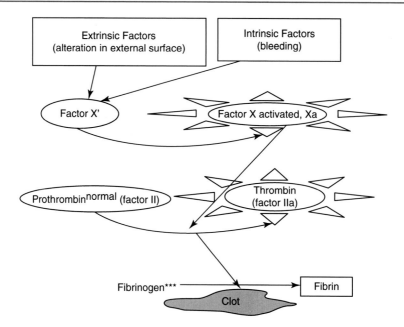

Fig. 5.1 Coagulation in ageing, a scheme.*,*** difference between young and old healthy donor. Thrombin and factor X activated are both targets of the new oral anticoagulants

the plasma proteins content in senescent-associated secretory phenotype, suggesting that the increased coagulation factors may have a CS SC origin—remember that coagulation factors are all proteases [40]. The pathophysiology of these abnormalities of coagulation factors is still unknown.

The pathophysiology of *colonic diverticular disease* is multifactorial. The disease is frequent and the formation of colonic diverticula increases with age [41]. Its pathophysiology is quite uncertain [42], and may be related either to a deficit in the regenerative capacities of gut epithelium from their stem cells or to alterations in the vast immune system linked to ageing ([33], see Sect. 5.3).

5.4 Biological Rhythms

The modifications of biological rhythms and more especially of the circadian rhythms was previously an exclusive physiological domain which is progressively becoming more molecular since the discovery of different genes referred as "clock controlled genes", present in nearly every tissue and every living species [43–45] (see Annex E). Ageing is associated with a disruption of circadian rhythmicity and reduces the amplitude and moves up the acrophase of most of the circadian variations (Table 5.2). Numerous physiological variables are concerned by this phenomenon such as sleep, body temperature, mood and cognitive acuity, cardiac, respiratory, and renal function, and most aspects of digestion and detoxification,

Table 5.2 Another seminal paper

In human beings, fibroblasts in a culture infected with a lentiviral bioluminescent circadian reporter, it is possible to reproducibly monitor the circadian oscillations of the cells and to measure their periods. In vitro fibroblast period lengths correlated with period lengths obtained in vivo in three different groups of young subjects. In addition, and not surprisingly, the authors found that average physiological period lengths were longer in blind subjects, nevertheless, interestingly, on average, blind individuals showed the same fibroblast clock properties as sighted ones. So human clock properties when measured in peripheral tissues, like dermal fibroblasts, mimic those measured more behaviorally in the same individual

The clock properties of human fibroblasts cultivated from dermal biopsies were further characterized in young and old persons. Interestingly, fibroblast period length, amplitude, and phase were unaltered in cells coming from older individuals, suggesting that the basic properties of the clocks of the elderly were not modified. Nevertheless, an important finding was made when young or old fibroblasts were incubated in the presence of serums. The serum from old persons significantly shortened the period length and advanced the phase of the circadian cellular rhythm, so far mimicking the in vivo situation. The serum factor responsible for this effect was a thermolabile factor, providing an ideal control for such experiments. One suggestion was that, in the elderly, less light exposure due, for example, to changes in lens properties would reduce the ability of light to entrain the central clock causing an ensuing fragmentation of the sleep/awake cycle, possibly in relation to hormonal status. Another possible explanation is that the senescent thermolabile factor was only specific to the central master clock

The secretome of human SCs can change the properties of the peripheral cellular clock [45, 46]

systolic arterial pressure, heart rate, urinary catecholamines excretion, and plasma renin, cortisol, aldosterone and melatonin concentrations. Recently, it was also suggested that the proteasome function is regulated by the circadian system [47]. Clock components remain nearly unaltered during aging; nevertheless, ageing is associated with tissue-specific rewiring, such as oscillation in protein acetylation, which can be prevented by calorie restriction [48, 49].

Sleep is under hypothalamic control and there is evidence that disruptions of the circadian rhythms parallel sleep disorders and fragmentation and neuronal degeneration, indicating a progressive deterioration of the circadian pacemaker with ageing. Ageing does not always bring about changes in sleep quantity. In healthy ageing subjects, the average sleeping time is around 6.5–7 h a day, but may cause changes in sleep architecture with an increased nighttime restlessness and daytime sleepiness, and a reduced amplitude of the sleep/awake rhythm (see, for example, Fig. 5 of [50] for the circadian rhythm in the number of arginine vasopressin-expressing neurons of the suprachiasmatic nucleus). For example, studies on young and elderly subjects under temporal isolation have reported a reduced amplitude and period of both body temperature and sleep/awake rhythms. This is accompanied by a change in the molecular responsiveness of the pacemaker to photic stimulation and a reduced expression of several genes encoding clock proteins. Nightly supplementation of melatonin was shown to improve sleep disorders, suggesting a potential therapeutic role for this hormone.

Rare studies have concerned *dreams* and dream recall in the elderly. Dream recall progressively decreases with age and this is attributed, in part, to sleeping disorders, especially the abnormalities in the rapid eye movement sleep period.

Patients suffering degenerative dementias are associated with a diminution of dreams, which may be linked to atrophy of sensory areas of the cortex [51].

The elderly presenting sleep disorders appear at a greater risk of mortality. With advancing age, the circadian cycles start to be disrupted, which indicates a progressive deterioration of the circadian pacemaker regulation during ageing. Obstructive sleep apnea increases in frequency with ageing, with prevalence rates as high as 60% above 60 years in certain meta-analysis. Involuntary, sometimes violent, movements may precede Parkinson's disease [50, 52]. Ageing is associated with a smoothing of most of the physiological rhythms, including the sleep/awake cycle, glycolysis, and calcium oscillations [53]. Heart rate is not regular and its irregularities are consequences of factors affecting vasomotricity, rheology, and age. The variations of arteriolar motricity are chaotic in behavior and under normal conditions, a dynamic structure of this type does not depend on pressure level since the correlation dimension remains unchanged at any level of cardiac flow, emphasizing that this property is an intrinsic property of the system. Conversely, the correlation dimension can be modified by pharmacologic manipulations. There are systems, like the sinus heart rate, which, under normal conditions, function with a linear dynamic and may shift to a chaotic behavior pattern using a strange attractor [54, 55].

The synthesis of *melatonin* is driven by several enzymes, and above all, by N-acetyl transferase, NAT, which is regulated and inhibited by light. The melatonin levels are 3–10 times higher during the nighttime than in the daytime in every living species and peak at 5 o'clock in the morning. Melatonin participates in the regulation of the circadian cycle, but it also has antioxidant properties. The effects of the hormone on lifespan are still debatable. Melatonin secretion and pineal NAT (during nighttime, from 8 to 1.5 nmol/gland/h) specific activity are strongly reduced in old rats and in old persons and may account, at least in part, for the sleeping disorders that are considered as a risk factor for several neurodegenerative diseases [56, 57, 58]. SCs could play a crucial role in the genesis of these alterations, but the topic is still poorly explored with one exception; Pagani et al. [45, 46] indeed showed that the clock properties of human fibroblasts in culture depended on a soluble secretome factor and were strongly attenuated in the presence of old animal plasma (summarized in Table 5.2). Krtolice et al. performed a similar experiment for cancer, see discussion in Sect. 6.1) [59].

Calorie restriction results in a rewiring of the circadian clocks. The demonstration was made on the transcriptome. The experimental demonstration is impressive; calorie restriction, indeed, significantly increases the number and amplitude of the expressions of circadian or oscillatory genes [48]. For a clinician the quality of sleep is mainly intuitively known, and there are, for the moment, very few systematic studies on this topic, except CALERIE 2, although the study was performed only in adults [60].

Thermoregulation is also a basic physiological function affected by ageing. It is strongly dependent on circadian clocks. The central temperature of the elderly and their resistance to extreme temperature variations are reduced (-0.4 °C). Also, during benign infections, fever is significantly attenuated in old persons [61, 62].

From a nearly ideological point of view, it is tempting to say, as did Lipsitz et al. [63], that life, health, and youth are linked to complexity, to nonlinear, to chaotic behavior and that, conversely, illness, senescence, the approach of death are accompanied by attenuated or irregular oscillations, meaning a dysregulation of our internal clocks. This is, for the moment, a declaration of principle, which requires factual confirmation. The frontier between stochastic and chaotic order is not self-evident [64, 65]—almost by definition—and we should remember that chaotic behavior is defined as an organization with the appearance of disorder. Nevertheless, the hypothesis "is supported by observations showing an age related loss of complex viability in multiple physiological processes" [63], while it can't be excluded that such a smoothing of these fluctuations may be a simple consequence of the decreased ability to exercise (see also "complexity" in Annex B).

Rhythmicity is a crucial property of life and is likely modified by the secretome of the SCs. Rhythmicity has to be understood before "treating" or preventing the clinical consequences of senescence.

5.5   The Senses and Sensitivity

Presbyacusis or age-related hearing loss reflects changes in both the peripheral and central auditory systems with an initial impact on the higher frequencies, which are the most important for understanding spoken language. Hearing loss in the elderly is independently associated with the development of cognitive decline and dementia. Much recent progress was made in improving hearing techniques based on stem cell progress [66, 67].

Uncorrected *presbyopia* is extremely frequent in ageing and represents a global burden of potential loss. It is commonly defined as a refractive condition in which the accommodative ability of the eye is insufficient for near vision, due to ageing [68]. The current hypothesis is that presbyopia is mainly due to an increased stiffening and viscoelasticity properties of the natural lens, which predominates in the nucleus and is not due to compaction of the lense nucleus. The lense has been proposed as an avascular and non-innervated model for fibrosis [69].

Cataract is a leading cause of age-related blindness worldwide. Age-related cataract lense constituents have many similar characteristics, especially for example, those concerning oxidation and the loss of antioxidants. Recently, several authors have involved lens proteostasis in the physiopathology of cataracts and insisted on the involvement of endoplasmic reticulum stress-induced unfolded protein response, age, and diabetes as being the most important risk factors. A considerable amount of cataractogenic stressors were identified and most of them can generate misfolded proteins of the membrane luminal and secretory proteins in the highly oxidized lumen of the endoplasmic reticulum. An unfolded protein response was described as a central determinant of the production of misfolded crystalline aggregation in the lens [70].

Impairments in *smell and taste* with ageing are widely overlooked and often neglected in geriatric practice. In contrast to taste, which is remarkably conserved with ageing, smell, olfaction decrease and anosmia is apparently linked to severe brain disorders [71]. There are data suggesting that taste disorder in the elderly was mainly linked to multiple medications that would impair the ability to taste the five basic flavors (salty, sweet, sour, bitter, and umami) [72].

Presbyalgesia The pressure pain thresholds of the head and neck muscles are higher in elderly subjects than in the young. This increased pain sensitivity was sometimes considered as an adaptive mechanism and is likely to reflect a central dysregulation [73, 74].

References

1. Ferrucci L, et al. Time and metrics of aging. Circ Res. 2018;123:740–4.
2. Naylor RM, et al. Senescent cells: a novel therapeutic target for aging and age-related diseases. Clin Pharmacol Ther. 2013;93:105–16.
3. Rittié L, et al. Natural and sun-induced aging of human skin. Cold Spring Harb Perspect Med. 2015;5:a015370.
4. Rodier F, Campisi J, et al. Four faces of cellular senescence. J Cell Biol. 2011;192:547–56.
5. Lönnqvist F, et al. Catecholamine-induced lipolysis in adipose tissue of the elderly. J Clin Invest. 1990;85:1614–21.
6. Camell CD, et al. Inflammasome-driven catecholamine catabolism in macrophages blunts lipolysis during ageing. Nature. 2017;550:119–23.
7. Tchkonia T, et al. Fat tissue, aging, and cellular senescence. Aging Cell. 2010;9:667–84.
8. Hemmatian H, et al. Aging, osteocytes, and mechanotransduction. Curr Osteoporos Rep. 2017;15:401–11.
9. Khosla S, et al. Inhibiting cellular senescence: a new therapeutic paradigm for age-relates osteoporosis. J Clin Endocrinol Metab. 2018;103:1282–90.
10. Pierce JL, et al. Defining osteoblast and adipocyte lineages inn the bone marrow. Bone. 2019;118:2–7. https://doi.org/10.1016/j.bone.2018.05.019.
11. Beaudart C, et al. Health outcomes of sarcopenia: a systematic review and meta-analysis. PLoS One. 2017;12:e0169548.
12. Drew L. Lifting the burden of old age. Nature. 2018;555:S15–7.
13. Eliazer S, et al. Cause and consequence in aged-muscle decline. Nature. 2016;540:349.
14. Piasecki M, et al. Failure to expand the motor unit size to compensate for declining motor unit numbers distinguishes sarcopenic from non-sarcopenic older men. J Physiol (Lond). 2018;596:1627–37.
15. Schwörer S, et al. Epigenetic stress responses induce muscle stem-cell ageing by Hox9 developmental signals. Nature. 2016;540:428.
16. Zhang G, et al. Hypothalamic programming of systemic aging involving IKK-β, NF-κB and GnRH. Nature. 2013;497:211–6.
17. Zhu J, et al. Genome-wide chromatin state transitions associated with developmental and environmental cues. Cell. 2013;152:642.
18. Hirschfeld HP, et al. Osteosarcopenia: where bone, muscle and fat collide. Osteoporos Int. 2017;28:2781–90.
19. Swynghedauw B. Developmental and functional adaptation of contractile proteins in cardiac and skeletal muscle. Physiol Rev. 1986;66:710–71.
20. Verdijk JB, et al. Satellite cells in human skeletal muscle; from birth to old age. Age. 2014;36:545–57.

21. Childs BG, et al. Senescent intimal foam cells are deleterious at all stages of atherosclerosis. Science. 2016;354:472–7.
22. Brondello JM, et al. Cellular senescence is a common characteristic shared by preneoplasic and osteo-arthritic tissue. Open Rheumatol J. 2010;4:10–4.
23. Jeon OH, et al. Local clearance of senescent cells attenuates the development of post-traumatic osteoarthritis and creates a pro-regenerative environment. Nat Med. 2017;23:775–82.
24. MacCulloch K, et al. Cellular senescence in osteoarthritis pathology. Aging Cell. 2017;16:210–8.
25. Fried L, et al. Frailty in older adults: evidence for a phenotype. J Gerontol A Biol Sci Med Sci. 2001;56:M146–56.
26. Rolland Y, et al. Frailty in older population: a brief position paper from the French society of geriatrics and gerontology. Geriatr Psychol Neuropsychiatr Vieil. 2011;9:387–90.
27. Begg DP. Disturbances of thirst and fluid balance associated with aging. Physiol Behav. 2017;178:28–34.
28. Panda A, et al. Human innate immunosenescence: causes and consequences for immunity in old age. Trends Immunol. 2009;30:325–33.
29. Shaw AC, et al. Aging of the innate immune system. Curr Opin Immunol. 2010;22:507–13.
30. Ergen AV, et al. Mechanisms of hematopoietic stem cell aging. Exp Gerontol. 2010;45:289–90.
31. Guralnik JM, et al. Prevelence of anemia in persons 65 years old and older in the US: evidence for a high rate of unexplained anemia. Blood. 2004;104:2263–8.
32. Zape JP, et al. Hemogenic endothelium: origins, regulation and implications for vascular biology. Semin Cell Dev Biol. 2011;22:1036–47.
33. Man AI, et al. The impact of aging on the intestinal epithelial barrier and immune system. Cell Immunol. 2014;289:112–8.
34. Ansell J. Bleeding in very old patients on vitamin K antagonist therapy. Circulation. 2011;124:768–71.
35. Gharacholou SM, et al. Hemostasis and thrombosis in older adults. J Thromb Thrombolysis. 2009;27:249–51.
36. Poli D, et al. Bleeding risk in very old patients on vitamin K antagonist treatment: results of a prospective collaborative study on elderly patients followed by Italian centres for anticoagulation. Circulation. 2011;124:824–9.
37. Capodanno D, et al. Antithrombotic therapy in the elderly. J Am Coll Cardiol. 2010;56:1683–92.
38. Franchini M. Hemostasis and agirng. Critical Rev Oncol Hematol. 2006;60:144–51.
39. Hager K, et al. Blood coagulation factors in the elderly. Arch Gerontol Geriatr. 1989;9:277–82.
40. Tanaka T, et al. Plasma proteomic signature of age in healthy humans. Aging Cell. 2018;17:e12799.
41. Camilleri M, et al. Insights into the pathophysiology and mechanisms of constipation, irritable bowel syndrome, and diverticulosis in older people. J Am Geriatr Soc. 2000;48:1142–50.
42. Burkhard HA, et al. Pathogenesis of colonic diverticular disease. Langenbeck's Arch Surg. 2012;397:1025–33.
43. Arellanes-Licea E, et al. The circadian timing system: a recent addition in the physiological mechanisms underlying pathological and aging process. Aging Dis. 2014;5:406–18.
44. Mure LS, et al. Diurnal transcriptome atlas of a primate across major neural and peripheral tissues. Science. 2018;359(6381):eaao0318. https://doi.org/10.1126/science.aao0318.
45. Pagani L, et al. The physiological period length of the human circadian clock in vivo is directly proportional to period in human fibroblasts. PLoS One. 2010;5(10):e13376.
46. Pagani I, et al. Serum factor in older individuals change cellular clock properties. Proc Natl Acad Sci U S A. 2011;108:7218–23.
47. Desvergne A, et al. Circadian modulation of proteasome activity and accumulation of oxidized protein in human embryonic kidney HEK 23 cells and primary derma fibroblasts. Free Radic Biol Med. 2016;4:195–207.
48. Hatanaka F, et al. Keeping the rhythm while changing the lyrics: circadian biology in aging. Cell. 2017;170:599–600.

49. Sato S, et al. Circadian reprogramming in the liver identifies metabolic pathways of aging. Cell. 2017;170:678–92.
50. Hofman MA, et al. Living with the clock: the circadian pacemaker in older people. Ageing Res Rev. 2006;5:33–51.
51. Guenole F, et al. Le rêve au cours du vieillissement normal et pathologique. Psychol Neuropsychiatr. 2010;8:87–96.
52. Sterniczuk R, et al. Sleep disturbances in older ICU patients. Clin Interv Aging. 2014;9:969–77.
53. Goldbeter A. Biochemical oscillations and cellular rhythms. The molecular bases of periodic and chaotic behaviour. Cambridge: Cambridge University Press; 1996.
54. LePape G, et al. Statistical analysis of sequences of cardiac interbeat intervals does not support the chaos hypothesis. J Theor Biol. 1997;184:123–31.
55. Yaniv Y, et al. The end effector of circadian heart variation: the sinoatrial node pace-maker. BMB Rep. 2015;48:677–84.
56. Touitou Y, et al. Modifications of circadian and circannual rhytthms with aging. Exp Gerontol. 1997;32:603–14.
57. Touitou Y. Human ageing and melatonin. Clinical relevance. Exp Gerontol. 2001;36:1083–100.
58. Cornelissen G, et al. Chronobiology of aging: a minireview. Gerontology. 2017;63:118–28.
59. Krtolica A, et al. Senescent fibroblasts promote epithelial cell growth and tumorigenesis: a link between cancer and aging. PNAS. 2001;98:12072–7.
60. Martin CK, et al. Effect of calorie restriction on mood, quality of life, sleep, and sexual function in healthy non-obese adults: the calerie 2 randomized clinical trial. JAMA Intern Med. 2016;176:743–52.
61. Blatteis CM. Age-dependent changes in thermoregulation. A mini review. Gerontology. 2012;58:289–95.
62. Weinert D. Circadian temperature variation and ageing. Ageing Res Rev. 2010;9:51–60.
63. Lipsitz LA, et al. Loss of "complexity" and aging. Potential applications of fractals and chaos theory to senescence. JAMA. 1992;267:1806–9.
64. Jasson S, et al. Instant power spectrum analysis of heart rate variability during orthostatic tilt using a time-frequency domain method. Circulation. 1997;96:3521–6.
65. Léger JJ, et al. From molecular to modular cardiology. How to interpret the million of data that came out from large scale analysis of gene expression? Arch Mal Coeur Vaiss. 2006;99:231–6.
66. Fortunato S, et al. A review of new insights on the association between hearing loss and cognitive decline in ageing. Acta Otorhinolaryngol Ital. 2016;36:155–66.
67. Patel R, et al. Hearing loss in the elderly. Clin Geriatr Med. 2018;34:163–74.
68. Charman WN. Virtual issue editorial: presbyopia – grappling with an age-old problem. Ophtalmic Physiol Opt. 2017;37:655–60.
69. Elred JA, et al. The lens as a model for fibrotic disease. Philos Trans R Soc Lond B Biol Sci. 2011;366:1301–19.
70. Periasamy P, et al. Age-related cataracts: role of unfolded protein response, Ca2+ mobilization, epigenetic DNA modifications, and loss of Nrf2/Keap1 dependent protection. Prog Retin Eye Res. 2017;60:1–19.
71. Mondon K, et al. Perception of tatse and smell in normal and pathological aging: an update. Geriatr Psychol Neuropsychiatr Vieil. 2014;12:313–20.
72. Imoscopi A, et al. Taste loss in the elderly: epidemiology, causes, and consequences. Aging Ciln Exp Res. 2012;24:570–9.
73. Marini I, et al. Aging effect on pressure thresholds of head and neck muscles. Aging Clin Exp Res. 2012;24:239–44.
74. Yezierski RP. The effects of age on pain sensitivity: preclinical studies. Pain Med. 2012;13(Suppl 2):S27–36.

Age-Linked Non-Transmissible Diseases

6

Abstract

Age-linked non-transmissible disease is becoming a new epidemiological category, which is likely to be mostly favored or even caused by the biological (in-) activity of senescent cells and their secretome.

Age is linked to several CNTD. However, the biological link and linking procedure between the two is not fully established for every disease; nevertheless, the causal effects of certain components of the senescent secretome are already documented for cancer, neurodegenerative diseases, and atherosclerosis. In addition, the regenerative capacity of the stem/progenitor cells in heart, kidney, pancreas, and lung diseases is progressively reduced, affecting the functioning of these organs.

The Chief Editor of the British Medical Journal (February 2018, see also [1]) pointed out recently that 50% of patients aged more than 60 years suffered from two associated diseases and this proportion is likely to reach nearly 80% after 80 years, concluding that it is urgent to include such types of multi diseases in medical teaching, and that it is also easy to predict that health costs will increase exponentially in future years (e.g., in the United States, in patients aged above 65, the cost of health care increased from $46,800 in 1970 to $145,000 in 1990). Based on a cohort of 418 patients, a population-based longitudinal study showed that multi morbidity has a higher incidence in old age and that mental health-related conditions were likely to be the best predictors of multi morbidity. The GBDS cohort [2–4] provided an important epidemiological basis; in 2017, the new medical landscape was radically modified, transmissible diseases were no more the major cause of mortality. All over the world, the major cause of mortality are CNTDs and this is a direct consequence of the globally increased prevalence of senescence [5, 6] (Table 6.1).

© Springer Nature Switzerland AG 2019

59

B. Swynghedauw, *The Biology of Senescence*, Practical Issues in Geriatrics,
https://doi.org/10.1007/978-3-030-15111-9_6

Table 6.1 The clinical manifestations of senescence: age-related diseases

- Cancers

- Neurodegenerative diseases (Parkinson's disease, amyotrophic lateral sclerosis, "dementias" including Alzheimer, vascular, mixed, frontotemporal and Lewy body dementias)

- Type 2 diabetes
- Obesity and fat dysfunction

- Clinical manifestations of atherosclerosis (stroke, myocardial infarction, peripheral arterial disease)
- Arterial hypertension
- Heart failure

- Renal failure
- Glomerulosclerosis

- Idiopathic pulmonary fibrosis
- Chronic obstructive pulmonary disease

- Age-related macular degeneration
- Glaucoma

6.1   Cancers

Like the roman god Janus [7], senescence also has two faces, on one side the anti-proliferative capacities of SCs have a beneficial role in tumor suppression and, probably, wound healing; nevertheless, the other side looks darker, the secretome of SCs strongly accelerates tissue proliferation [7], or, better, the Yin and Yang, the all good and the all bad (symbolized by the Japanese symbol, the *taijitu*). These two faces are interdependent and complementary identities and they both carry the seed of the other. Senescence favors cancer but, this is obviously not the only factor involved, lung cancer is more frequent at 65 years than at 90 [8] (see Fig. 2.1), but the prognosis is much better in a rich person than in a poor one. Conversely, experimentally, the components of senescence have been used to treat cancer and several papers have been published with encouraging results.[1] Several clinicians may also have experienced that certain cancers have a better prognosis in very old persons, although this population appears as being quite heterogeneous. Accordingly, a study based on a cohort of 803 patients, mean age 72 years, showed, in older adults with cancer, that certain geriatric parameters (cognitive impairment) were associated with shorter survival after hospitalization [10].

The main cellular process at the origin of senescence is a blockade of cell regeneration; in contrast, cancer is the result of an accelerated and uncontrolled local cell proliferation and the relevance of senescence for cancer protection has been frequently evoked (Table 6.2). Moreover, it is also clear that cancers are very significantly more frequent in old persons than in adults; this two-sided aspect of pathological senescence is a crucial clinical problem [11–13]. To add to the

---

[1] For example, there is evidence that in an oncogene induced model of cancer, senescence will limit the progression of the process [7].

Table 6.2 The roman god Janus paradox opposing senescent and cancer cells

	Senescent cell	Cancer cell
Cellular proliferation	⇓	⇑
Genome instability		⇑
Telomere and telomerase	Shortening of telomeres with telomerase inhibition	Shortening of telomeres but telomerase activation
Epigenetic alterations	– DNA hypomethylation – miR 17–92 down regulation	Complicated, depends on the gene regulated
Proteostasis	Impaired	Augmented
Stem cells	Exhausted	May be a nidus for tumorigenesis

complexity, cell ageing and stem cell ageing are driven by multiple and diverse cell-intrinsic mechanisms, including the unavoidable accumulation of DNA mutations and replication errors that are major components of cancer etiology [14]. The pathophysiology of cancer is a complicated issue that associates two evolutionary antagonistic phenomena[2]: the survival of cancer cells notwithstanding the individual finality and the survival of the whole individual [12, 13, 21 22], the roman god Janus paradox [7] (Table 6.2).

Increased telomere shortening is a well-documented finding during ageing. Accelerated telomere shortening may be related to cancer incidence by increasing chromosomal instability. However, the relationships between telomere length and cancer etiology were rather inconsistent. In a large longitudinal cohort study with similar age (A cohort of 792 participants of the Normative Aging Study, NAS, from the US Department of Veterans Affairs, with a follow-up between 1992 and 2012), the age-related blood telomere length attrition was faster in cancer cases pre-diagnosis than in cancer-free patients; the age-adjusted telomere length attrition began decelerating as diagnosis approached, resulting in longer telomere length 3–4 years prior to diagnoses of cancer. This could explain the previous inconsistencies. The longitudinal nature of this study enabled the authors to confirm the decline in telomere length with age and to establish temporal associations between telomere length and cancer incidence [21, 23].

The cellular senescence concept states that the development of cancer cells requires a particular environment like the secretome of the SCs. This hypothesis is also supported by the fact that some tumor cells possess mutations,[3] which inhibit the SC program [12]. A convincing paper has been published by Krtolica et al. [24] (summarized in Table 6.3) who found that senescent human fibroblasts stimulate

---

[2] See Table 6.2 and the different papers that were periodically published after Stratton's paper on the hallmarks of cancer [15–17]. One of the major problems that arose from these articles was that senescence itself was usually seen as a factor, like genome instability, and not as a conglomerate similar to the various conglomerates at the origins of cancer.

[3] At the level of Trp53 or of CDKN-2alpha.

Table 6.3 A seminal paper

Early in life, cellular senescence which is an arrest of proliferation appears to be a major barrier against progress to malignancies and certain evidence suggests that senescence response inhibits tumorigenesis, and senescent fibroblasts stimulate and facilitate preneoplastic and neoplastic epithelial growths while they do not have any effect on the normal growth of normal epithelial cells. This activation is largely linked to the creation of a microenvironment that facilitates the progression of the mutant cells and is linked to the secretion of diffusible soluble or insoluble factors secreted by the SCs. In cell culture, growth stimulation was observed when 10% of the fibroblast population was made by senescent fibroblasts

Senescent fibroblasts promote epithelial cell growth and tumorigenesis [24]

premalignant and malignant epithelial cells to proliferate in culture and form tumors in mice. For Krtolica, "although cellular senescence suppresses tumorigenesis early in life, it may promote cancer in aged organisms, suggesting that this was an example of evolutionary antagonistic pleiotropy" (see Sect. 8.1, Tables 6.1 and 6.3, and Annex B).

Several papers also confirmed this property for senescent fibroblasts, which was also attributed to several soluble factors of the secretome like VEGF, different MMPs, amphiregulin; some of these factors may explain resistance to chemotherapy [25]. Several other arguments reinforce these findings, including the fact that, experimentally, senescent fibroblasts and the presence of certain metalloproteases in their secretome disrupt the breast tissue morphogenesis and milk production. Several miRs play a role in the diffusion of metastasis [26]. Cancer and senescence have genome instability in common, but not at the same location on the genome, it's not a "property", it generates de facto multiple mutations whose effects may, by accident, block or, conversely, activate proliferation[4] [12, 14, 27–31]. Luck has nothing to do with any result, biology, evolutionary biology is firstly the result of a general tinkering process [32].

6.2   Neurodegenerative Diseases

Two recent Insight/Outlook articles in the publication Nature were on neurodegenerative diseases.[5] Heemels's editorial in Nature Insight outlines the fact that these diseases are not only linked to ageing. In this issue, an updated article summarizes the prion hypothesis in Parkinson's disease (Nature Insight, 2016, 539, 179). Neurodegenerative diseases include a large group of affections, which, in fact, have clinically very little in common except that they usually happen in old persons, have a neurocerebral origin with a poor therapeutic approach, and a pathophysiology still largely hypothetical but mainly centered around the framework of proteinopathies [33]. Neurodegenerative diseases include the various forms of

---

[4] Numerous oncogenes, with sometimes opposite functions, are involved in this process and also a group of seven proteins which stabilize the genome, the sirtuin family.

[5] The readers who would like to explore the pathophysiology of AD more in depth are invited to consult these two remarkable issues.

dementia—Alzheimer's disease, AD, the Lewy body, frontotemporal and vascular dementias, amyotrophic lateral sclerosis, and Parkinson's disease (Table 2.4). Their incidence parallels the increasing mean age of the population. For dementias, both the nosological framework and diagnosis criteria are still a problem so that the exact diagnosis which is recorded on the official death registers is usually "dementia" or even "Alzheimer's," with no real diagnosis criteria. In addition, there are many cases in which two types of dementia are associated, the most frequent being the association of vascular and Alzheimer dementia.

More recently, Richard Hodson, supplement editor of Nature, reached a similar conclusion and added a fairly depressing comment (Nature Outlook on Alzheirmer's disease 2018, 559, S1–S18). He said that "despite decades of research, there are still no drugs that can slow down the progression of AD, let alone offer a cure. Promised preclinical results have repeatedly failed to translate into treatments for people. The hypothesis that amyloid-beta deposits in the brain cause AD is now under great pressure to deliver an effective therapy, and the desire to explore alternative approach is growing".

To increase the complexity of the problem, it is now well-established that the existence of cerebrovascular problems may aggravate AD by slowing the elimination of amyloid substances. Weller et al. [34] have shown in a group of AD patients that thromboembolic occlusion of cortical arteries affects the distribution of the amyloid substance beta. Early deposition of the amyloid substance beta was related to individual arterial territories in the brain and that there is an inverse relationship between capillary amyloid angiopathy and plaques of amyloid substance beta. The epidemiological data are frequently confusing and difficult to interpret [34–36].

A seminal review article, based on data from the multi-generational, community-based Framingham study summarized the most important clinical data from a pathophysiological point of view [37]. The follow-up of the Framingham cohort starts in 1976 and was based on both cognitive and imaging testing, including a battery of neuropsychological tests and, since 1999, magnetic resonance imaging, MRI. The frequency of AD was correlated with several risk factors. (1) Heritability is high, multigenic, and correlated to several genetic variants, as ApoE epsilon 4, the sortilin receptor, the retinal cadherin and several others [38, 39]. (2) The disease is associated with high levels of docohexaenoic acid (DHA), homocystein, and diabetes. (3) AD, like diabetes, is associated with a low level inflammatory state with a significant elevation of various blood cytokines [40]. (4) Finally, there is a significant correlation with a hyper-intensity signal on MRI and clinical signs, the MRI signals preceding the clinical signs.

The diagnosis criteria are regularly reevaluated, and they now include the clinical criteria (including anosognosia), imaging (MRI, PET, and SPECT) [41], and several biomarkers (decreased beta amyloid substance and increased total tau protein and phospho tau in the cerebrospinal fluid and the presence of amyloid protein or its fragments in the plasma) [42–45]. Bousiges and Blanc [46] have recently proposed as markers for AD and Lewy bodies dementia, the following: total tau protein, phosphorylated tau $_{181}$, Abeta 42 and Abeta 40 in the cerebrospinal fluid. It is now possible to have a high degree of confidence in the early stages of the disease, which opens up new therapeutic perspectives.

The neuro degeneratives have, for the moment, comparable pathophysiological mechanisms. Ageing, obviously, is an important factor at the origin of neuronal degenerescence. Moreover, no doubt protein homeostasis—proteostasis—is also involved and this is still an incompletely explored mechanism (not only for cerebral tissue, but also for the heart (see Sect. 6.5.1) and the accompanying figures). The phenomenon is likely to be accelerated by a combination of genetic and environmental factors.

Pathological studies, at present, support the general hypothesis that the accumulation of misfolded aggregated proteins in the brain are the trigger of a complicated series of events that finally result in neuronal degeneration and the clinical evidence of an AD ([47], see Sects. 3.4 and 4.2). Among the different and multiple findings evidenced to date, there are a few morphological abnormalities, which were, currently, commonly considered as hallmarks of AD, namely, the accumulation of both amyloid beta-peptide, Abeta, deposits in the form of plaques and neurofibrillar tangles made of hyperphosphorylated tau protein. In addition, a recent meta-analysis has reported neuronal and synaptic loss linked to the severity of the cognitive impairment [48, 49]. SC play a causal role in the genesis of tau-mediated diseases. Bussian et al. [47] were using a transgenic mouse model expressing high levels of tau proteins in neurons with the development of neurofibrillar tangle deposition starting in hippocampus and neurodegeneration and cognitive disorders. These mice have high levels of SC. Transgenic manipulation was utilized to suppress these SC. The suppression of SC in astrocytes and microglia, but not in neurons, prevents the hyperphosphorylation of tau proteins and preserve cognitive functions. Conversely, there also are strong suggestions that tau proteins themselves may induce SC.

Adult neural stem/progenitor cells, NSPC, reside in a few brain regions such as the mediobasal *hypothalamic region* and the sub-ventricular zone of the lateral ventricle in the brain, which mediate local neurogenesis and several aspects of cerebral functioning. NSPC has been identified by using several biomarkers, including, for example, a nuclear transcription factor, Sox2. The mediobasal hypothalamus is crucial for neuroendocrine regulation. The concentration in NSPC diminishes with age and the experimental ablation of NSPC (using a viral mediobasal hypothalamic injection) shows ageing-like physiological decline and reduces lifespan. Their implantation slowed down ageing (as measured with various physiological parameters: muscle endurance, coordination, treadmill performance, sociality, and novel object recognition) and increased lifespan. Modulation of the ageing process by NSPC was observed in a relatively short period lasting 3–4 months. NSPC secretes a large amount of exosomal miRs as compared to other regions of the hypothalamus and treatment with these exosomes slows down ageing. Clearly, the NSPC have a programmatic role in systemic ageing, acting both through their endocrine function and neurogenesis [50].

Presently, there is a rather large consensus around a crucial disorder in the regulation of the metabolism of the precursor of the beta-amyloid protein, which is normally present in the brain and accumulates with ageing to form amyloid plaques, the amyloid cascade (Fig. 3.4). The beta-amyloid protein is a well-characterized peptide of 40–42 amino acids [51], resulting from a cleavage driven by two specific proteases. Such an accumulation precedes the development of neurofibrils and that of the cognitive deficit, and is responsible for the accumulation of a toxic protein, the tau protein [52]. Phosphorylation of the tau protein entails neurofibrillar dege-neresence, which finally will kill the neuronal cells [53]. Golde et al. [54] and Venegas et al. [40] have proposed an integrative hypothesis based on recognition of the amyloid substance as non-self and, as such, as a chronic astrocytes activator of the immune system.

Senescent astrocytes have been evidenced in the brain of patients suffering from AD and also in old persons without the symptoms of AD, which is in favor of the role of SC as a determinant of neurodegenerative diseases. Zhang et al. [50] unambiguously demonstrated that the adult neural stem/progenitor cells of the hypothalamus are a major determinant in the senescence process. The secretome of these cells is extremely rich in pro-inflammatory factors (above all, the inter-leukin, IL6). In addition, a beta-amyloid substance, like hypoxia, has a pro-ageing effect and may induce the expression of the same senescent biomarkers as those existing in human astrocytes [54, 55]. There is much data favoring the role of the inflammatory pathways (like IL-1alpha) in the formation of beta-amyloid peptide in AD. These inflammatory factors are present in the microvesicles secreted by the SC of the central nervous system. These vesicles were also found in the amy-loid plaques and may be used as markers of the disease as well as several miRs [50, 56–59].

For the moment, trials focused on the amyloid hypothesis have yielded negative results and other different hypotheses have been proposed concerning the patho-physiology of the disease. The prion hypothesis is one of the most popular. The figures published in Nature by Jucker and Walker [60] support this hypothesis, which states that "proteinaceous seeds" could be the self-propagating agents for the instigation and progression of neurodegenerative diseases. The specific protein-aceous lesions adopt an amyloid conformation and show a prion-like self-propaga-tion and spreading consistent with the progressive diffusion over time of the lesions, amyloid plaques, and neurofibrillar structure (rich in tau substance) in the brain of patients with AD, alpha synuclein I, body Lewy dementia, or inclusions of TDP-43 in the medulla motoneurones of the lateral amyotrophic sclerosis. As a strong support to the prion hypothesis, it was shown that the amyloid beta protein was inducible in the brain by the injection of extract into the intraperitoneal cavity and that the disease can be transmitted by injecting human proteinaceous substances into mice [54, 60].

The infectious hypothesis was reviewed in detail by Itzhaki et al. [61] who sug-gests an entry of bacteria or other infectious agents through the olfactory system. The hypothesis was recently rejuvenated by the discovery of the herpes virus in the brains of patients with AD [62].

Autophagy is a well-regulated physiological process in charge of purifying the useless proteins, including aggregates or unfolded peptides. Autophagy slows with ageing, contributing to the accumulation of abnormal or unfolded proteins. In addition, the expression of several genes controlling autophagy, such as *atg5* and *atg7*, is reduced with ageing. In experimental models, the activation of autophagy significantly increases the lifespan [54, 63].

Another hypothesis proposed that AD belongs to the autoimmune diseases. This hypothesis is supported by epidemiological data and by the fact that incidence of the disease is negatively correlated with the microbial environment [64].

Several environmental toxics have been accused of, at least, favoring the appearance of certain neurodegenerative diseases. The most documented are pesticides used in agriculture and the Parkinson's disease. The relative risk of developing an AD or a Parkinson's in old people exposed for professional reasons was measured in France in a cohort of 1507 subjects, and was, respectively, 5.63 and 2.39, which is high [65, 66].

Hundreds of therapeutic trials have been performed so far, with, currently, no positive results for clinical purposes, very likely "too little too late" [67]. Some of these trials were based on interesting pathophysiological concepts like, for example, that of Bredesen [68]. This author assumes the existence of a metabolic disorder and suggests that most of the therapeutic failures were due to either the absence of any dietetic correction or to the fact that the treatment was started too late. Information from the EU-US CTAD Task Force concerning the amyloid-targeting drugs are still negative and support the consensus that any effective drug therapy requires intervention in the early, even pre-symptomatic stages of the disease and other hypotheses than the amyloid hypothesis should be explored [69].

6.3   Type 2 Diabetes and Metabolic Syndrome

The massive increased incidence of type 2 diabetes in old persons is the result of the combination of at least two different factors, the decrease in the regenerative capacities of the beta Langerhans cells of the pancreas, which become SCs (see Sect. 4.2, Fig. 4.2and Table 4.2) and a group of factors that enhance insulin resistance (Table 6.4) [72].

Insulin resistance causes compensatory proliferation of the pancreatic Langerhans beta cells that have a limited proliferative capacity and a low turnover [72]. Both chronic hyperglycemia and hyperlipidemia exert deleterious effects on the beta cells, the first being a prerequisite for the toxicity of the second consistent with the clinical observation that the majority of hyperlipidemic patients are not diabetic [73, 74]. The corresponding clinical experience is the frequent necessity of modifying diabetes treatment with ageing, and of shifting the treatment to insulin after a certain age.

Older patients are at risk of the development of type 2 diabetes as a result of the combined effects of lifestyle, genetic and ageing influence. Age is associated with multiple components that facilitate the onset of diabetes: insulinoresistance, overweight, and sedentarity. An enhanced activation of "nutrient sensing" pathways with age has been reported and may contribute to insulin resistance" [75].

Table 6.4 Diabetes and senescence

Diminution of the pancreatic beta cells (reduction of the regeneration capacity of the cells), insulin secretion in response to glucose is also reduced

Diminution of insulin resistance due to a combination of
- Inflammatory factors of the secretome
- Reduction of physical activity
- Obesity
- Multiple comorbidities (arterial hypertension, cognitive impairments) or their medications (glucocorticoids)
- Genetic factors: At least 60 variants [70]

Elevated plasma glucose per se causes CV disease. (1) the advanced glycated end product receptor activation is responsible for an increased intima-medial thickening and the consecutive augmented arterial stiffness. (2) Hyperglycemia stimulates the arterial formation of macrophages and of foam cells and (3) promotes the oxidative stress and the consecutive fibrosis. Obesity plays a major role in the pathogenesis of glucose metabolism dysfunction [71]

Adiponectin, an insulin sensitizer with anti-inflammatory properties, which is secreted by the adipose tissue also plays a role; nevertheless, this property is not yet fully documented in ageing (see, for example [76]). The influence of the metabolic factor in senescence is complex and not easily summarized. Studies in humans and rodents have evidenced that ageing exerts a distinct influence on beta cell turnover (which is low in adults) and function (see Barzilai et al. [77], Sone et al. [78], and Lee et al. [72]). Regeneration and proliferation of the beta Langerhans cells is a well-documented mechanism which adapts the pancreas to demand, this property is attenuated with ageing and is one of the first diabetogenic factors both in human and in experimental models [78].

Adiposity increases with ageing in human beings and in rats. With age, subcutaneous fat is reduced and visceral fat increases [77]. This very common clinical observation has many endocrine consequences and accounts for insulinoresistance. In experimental models, the ablation of fat restores insulinosensitivity. Adipose tissue is enriched in inflammatory factors (see Sect. 5.1 on immunometabolism, the major review article from [79]) and is de factor second risk factor). Glucose homeostasis is a fairly fragile function in humans and with ageing glucose progressively becomes a toxic nutrient [80].

6.4   Lungs, Kidneys and Liver Diseases

Lungs are modified during normal ageing. (1) Both the alveolar volume and the alveolar and bronchiolar conducts diameters are increased and bronchioles are frequently ectasic. (2) Alveolar and bronchiolar walls are thickened and less elastic. (3) Pulmonary capillary density is reduced. These are also aggravated by prolonged tobacco smoking. SCs—either epithelial, alveolar or fibroblastic—are common in old lungs [81]. The senescent fibroblasts play a particular role in the incidence of ageing on IPF, COPD, and emphysema [82] (Fig. 6.1). IPF is significantly associated, in human beings, with the presence of SCs (identified with the beta-galactosidase-p16, as a marker), whose abundance is in proportion to the

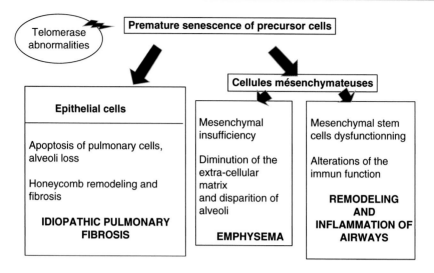

Fig. 6.1 The hypothesis of premature senescence as a cause of IPF and emphysema. The hypothesis postulates a premature senescence of epithelial or mesenchymal lung stem cells at the origin of these two diseases. Biological mechanisms are complex but well-documented and include telomerase activity and, for the secretome, the miRs. The two mechanisms, the epithelial and the mesenchymal, are combined when the two diseases are clinically associated (rearranged with data from [82])

severity of the disease, and in mice the transgenic suppression of these SCs significantly improves the lung function [83, 84].

Renal tissue is also modified with ageing. The kidney function is first affected by the proliferation of SCs. The reduction of the renal function with age is aggravated by tubular atrophy, the loss of nephrons with a compensatory hypertrophy of the remaining nephrons, interstitial fibrosis, and tubular diverticula. Glomerulosclerosis, which is the most frequent severe manifestation of renal senescence is a form of fibrosis linked to age. It has experimentally been shown that the ablation of SCs can improve, and even correct, the glomerular function and that glomerulosclerosis may be reversible [85]. After 30 years of age, it was estimated that a normal individual loses about 6000–6500 nephrons every year; nevertheless, the glomerular filtration is, in part, compensated for by the compensatory hypertrophy of the remaining nephrons [86]. With ageing, there is a reduction in the number of nephrons with compensatory hypertrophy of the remaining nephrons· and a decrease in capillary density associated with interstitial fibrosis. Tubular cells, which are extremely energy dependent, become more vulnerable to stress. Numerous elements of the renal SCs secretome participate in the process and are lead to age-linked kidney fibrosis [5, 85, 86].

In the *liver*, experimental data has suggested that, paradoxically, senescence may reduce fibrosis induced by activating several proteases and could facilitate the regression of cirrhosis after the arrest of the initial toxic process [87].

6.5 The Senescent CV System

In human beings and in experimental models, senescence is associated with several CV disorders.

- Normal ageing is said to be physiological, and it is accompanied by a specific CV phenotype, which is a direct consequence of the presence of SCs and of their secretome.
  - An old myocardium is different from an adult myocardium and senescence itself is responsible for several cellular (proteostasis) and extracellular (fibrosis) disorders, which account for the alterations of diastolic and systolic functions and also for changes in conduction properties, including in atria [88–94].
  - Vascular senescence is mainly characterized by an increase in the characteristic impedance of the large arteries and the ensuing impedance overload of the LV [95].
  - Senescent myocardial fibroblasts and vascular smooth muscle cells have a specific secretome that contains factors regulating cardiocyte proliferation, such as integrin beta 1, and genes associated with osteoblasts that account for calcifications of the media. Coronary artery calcium is a useful risk factor, even in the elderly, and the use of coronary calcification allows clinicians to reclassify risk even in the elderly. The biological explanation is the presence of osteoblasts from the SCs secretome [96–98].
- Pathological ageing is associated with several CV diseases as clinical CV manifestations of atherosclerosis or diabetes (Fig. 6.2).

6.5.1 The Senescent Myocardium

The senescent myocardium differs from a young one from both a functional and a biological view point, and there is evidence that adult cardiocytes are SCs and have lost their capacity to divide early in life (revue in [16, 99]). The present problem from both a clinical and a basic point of view is to know whether there are sufficient arguments to clearly identify senescent heart failure and to understand the mechanism that has driven this issue (Table 6.5).

From a Functional Point of View
1. The senescent LV is hypertrophied, and this hypertrophy does only concern the LV and is attributed to the impedance overloading and results from the increased impedance of the large arterial vessels created by the senescent-induced increase in the rigidity of these vessels [95] (see Sects. 6.5.2 and 6.5.3). The diastolic filling time progressively diminishes with age and this is the result of the progressive fibrosis of the ventricles (which is reflected by modifications of the E wave

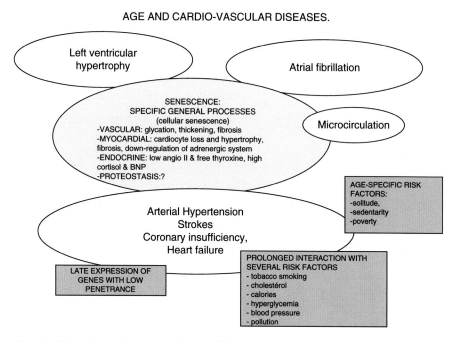

Fig. 6.2 The relations between ageing and CV diseases are a complicated issue. The general process of senescence is obviously predominant. Nevertheless, the retarded expression of many genes has also been clearly demonstrated, and obviously the present list needs to be completed. Above all, it is easy to understand that ageing is associated with a prolonged contact with a number of risk factors and also with several societal risks such as isolation or poverty. The latter may be predominant but are frequently difficult to evaluate

Table 6.5 Is the senescent heart a failing heart?

A failing heart, meaning a heart with a normal coronary vasculature, normal valves, and normal arterial pressure; there are numerous arguments favoring a progressive decline in cardiac function caused by the progressive senescence of the cardiocytes and their limited capacity to regenerate ([15], see [16] for the whole references)

From a clinical and physiological point of view, during ageing
- there are major defects in the diastolic function with dominant increased myocardial stiffness
- exercising is associated with a reduced ejection fraction and a normal sinus node response
- there is an age-related LV hypertrophy, which compensates for both the loss of cardiocytes and the characteristic impedance LV overload
- there are numerous arguments in favor of the senescent heart being a manifestation of HFpEF

From an experimental point of view, experiments with 28-month-old rats showed
- these animals are failing with a doubling of the tele-diastolic pressure and a strong depression of contractility in the papillary muscle

From a pathophysiological point of view
- fibrosis is mainly compensatory but also likely to be reactive. Ageing, with a normal coronary system, combines myocardial fibrosis due to the ageing process (the SCs secrete fibrogenic and proinflammatory factors) with a mechanical overload and depressed contractility at the molecular level
- Proteostasis abnormalities are likely to be the missing link that would explain the state of the senescent myocardium. An Alzheimer's heart has yet to be characterized [17]

at echo, which can now be measured using NMR) and the alteration of the reduction in calcium movement in the sarcoplasmic reticulum. The compensatory mechanism is an increased atrial contraction and an increase of the A wave. Such a diastolic dysfunctioning is one of the major characteristics of the senescent myocardium.

2. At rest, in old persons, cardiac output is normal and does not change with ageing, provided the subjects have normal coronary arteries. The Baltimore Longitudinal Study of Ageing [100] is a seminal work that includes several solid arguments concerning the normality of the coronary state, including stress and thallium test. It is indeed crucial in these approaches to eliminate any possibility of a latent ischemia since sensitivity to ischemia is increased by ageing [101]. During ageing, the most characteristic alteration is a reduced $VO2_{max}$ associated with a reduced ejection fraction. Old persons also have a reduced response to catecholamines and, during exercise, they increase their cardiac output, not by accelerating heart rate but by using the Starling law and increasing the ejection fraction [89–91].

3. The rat is a particular mammalian model because rats never spontaneously suffer from atheroma. The 28-month-old rat is the equivalent of a 80–85 year old human (rat mortality is around 70% at 28 months). Two different papers using this model have consistently shown that age was associated with a progressive deterioration of both systolic and diastolic functions [102, 103]. A major additional work from Rozenberg et al. [92] combined a hemodynamic study of contractility both in vivo and in vitro, on an isolated heart, with an analysis of both the papillary muscle and skinned fiber (ventricular muscle fibers without membrane) contractility. The authors evidenced a progressive degradation of systolic and diastolic functions, mainly due to ventricular fibrosis. Old rats have a 35% LV hypertrophy, a severe reduction of the systolic function (the systolic pressure is 131 mmHg in young animals and falls to à 108 at 28 months; the Vmax of papillary muscles falls from 3.76 to 2.16 L_{max} per sec), the LV diastolic compliance is also strongly modified (the chamber compliance, Kc, is 52 mL^{-1} in young animals and increasesto 99 in old animals), and, above all, they observed a pronounced elevation of the tele-diastolic pressure (from 4.8 to 7.9 mmHg). These very old animals, with a normal coronary circulation, are clearly experiencing heart failure, with a near doubling of their tele-diastolic pressure.

4. Finally, we must not forget the valvular diseases due to calcifications, which accumulate with ageing (especially aortic stenosis). The secretome of the senescent endothelial cells contains genes associated with osteoblasts, which are likely to be the origin of valvular and myocardial age-linked calcifications [96].

From a Biological Point of View

1. Adult cardiocytes have lost their capacity to divide and *stricto sensu* adult cardiocytes are already senescent, at least in part [16, 31, 99, 104–109]. In humans and in animals, the number of cardiac myocytes diminishes progressively with age, but, from a physiological point of view, this diminution is compensated for by a compensatory hypertrophy of the remaining cardiocytes. The molecular

stigmats of this compensatory hypertrophy are the same as we previously discovered in mechanical overload [110–112]. The same phenomenon exists in the kidney and lungs (Sect. 6.4).

2. The senescent cardiac cell is associated with increased oxidative stress and a reduction of leucocyte telomeres, which is, at the least, a biological proof of the general process of senescence. So, telomere length can also be viewed as a CV risk biomarker. Proteins that regulate telomerase activity are likely to have other properties than the regulation of telomere length. It has been suggested that these other properties are likely to explain the link between telomere length and the CV risk [113, 114]. Recently, the Athanase Benetos group suggested that a higher attrition rate of leukocyte telomere length in early life can modify the risk and timing of developing atherosclerosis [115]. The telomere length of endothelial stem cells and leucocytes has a prognosis value in coronary diseases. Six different studies, including the Framingham cohort, reached the same conclusion.

3. The senescent heart is fibrotic for several reasons [16, 92, 110, 111, 116, 117]. In contrast to other tissues [103], adult cardiocytes have lost their capacity to regenerate and continue to be progressively destroyed by apoptosis and ischemia [16]. Nevertheless, there are more and more "holes" in this tissue which are progressively filled with the inert fibrotic tissue. In addition, the senescent heart is often ischemic and also more sensitive to ischemia than the young heart [101, 119], the result is the presence of both a replacement and a reactive fibrosis. The fibrosis induced by the fibrogenic factors present in the SCs secretomes must be added to the list.

Fibrosis, even excessive or inappropriated replacement fibrosis, has many deleterious clinical consequences: it enhances diastolic stiffness and is the main constituent of diastolic dysfunction [16, 120, 121]. The stiffness of the collagen fiber, the thickening of the collagen layer, and, probably more, the nonalignment of collagen fibers with regard to the sarcomeres will disturb both the passive diastolic filling and the systolic ejection. To this well-known set of data, it is important to add abnormalities of the torsion of the myocardium—the "mop" effect—initially discovered by Torrent-Guasp [122–124]. Fibrous tissue is also an electrical isolator that will hamper electrical transmission and create re-entrees.

4. Proteostasis is a major biological component of cell homeostasis (Sect. 3.4), more especially in the myocardium, which is a syncytium and has to function as a whole without fail. So, cardiocyte functioning depends on tight control of synthesis, correct folding, lysis, and elimination of the lytic debris of proteins. Misfolded proteins and various protein debris are toxic for the cardiac, as well for the cerebral cell. Recently, several papers have strongly suggested that proteostasis abnormalities exist in the senescent and/or failing heart analogous to what has been reported in the Alzheimer's brain, and some authors have said that there is a "cardiac Alzheimer" [17, 125]. The cardiac content in HSPs could be considered as a sort of proxy for proteostasis. Several HSPs are elevated not only in the senescent heart but also in diabetic cardiopathy, after a myocardial

infarction or in atrial fibrillation. It is also associated with a low level inflammatory state, and a fall in the autophagic and proteostatic process[126]. Many mutations may modify the proteostatic process and cause cardiomyopathy [17, 127], the best documented concerns BAG3, which is a co-chaperone molecule. Inactivation of BAG3 results in dilated cardiomyopathy in mice [128]. The inactivation is reversible and the overexpression of FOXO can correct these abnormalities and restore the cardiac function [129].

At present, very few studies have focused on the relationships between proteostasis and myocardial function [125] (see chapter the origins of aging, section proteostasis). To function as a syncytium, the myocardium requires absolute control of protein homeostasis; the accumulation of misfolded proteins is toxic for the myocardial function and these proteins need correct refolding or recycling (Fig. 3.3). A transgenic-induced desmin-related cardiomyopathy has been described and is related to the accumulation of toxic amyloidosis products; but, currently, this is not documented in humans [130]. A work by Damien Logeart [131] has shown the existence of unexplained, nonischemic, cardiolysis in a group of heart failure patients aged over 65. Kostin [132] has also shown the heterogeneity of the autolytic cardiac mechanisms. In the same line, we may remember that Baker [133] also demonstrated that the destruction of SCs prevents compensatory cardiac cell hypertrophy in old mice (Table 4.1).

The most abundant of the HSPs in the heart is HSPB5 (also called alphaB-cristalline, CryAB). Myosin, an important constituent of any muscle, utilizes a specific chaperone for making its secondary and tertiary structures, UNC-45 [134]. The elimination of proteic debris is totally absent in certain desminopathies, and also severely hampered in old persons where it contributes to the cellular accumulation of toxic peptides. The physiological consequences of the accumulation of toxic debris on myocardial function is not yet fully documented; nevertheless, this is one of the best hypotheses for elucidating the pathogenesis of senescent cardiac dysfunction [17].

5. Senile systemic amyloidosis is characterized by the deposit of transthyretin-based amyloid substance in parenchymal organs, mainly within the heart, with heart failure and arrhythmias, in very old persons. A systematic autopsy study of 256 persons aged 85 or over has evidenced a high prevalence in this population (approximately 25% of people aged 85 or over and a strong association with myocardial infarction and several genetic variants in genes coding alpha2 macroglobulin and tau protein, suggesting that this well-known disease condition may be associated with amyloid deposition. The diagnosis is not easy and is generally an autopsy finding [135].

6.5.2   The Senescent Vascular System

The Arterial System
During ageing in human beings, the morphology of the arteries is modified: (1) both the diameter (from 6.9 cm between 19 and 44 years for the aortic cross to 8.5 cm

after 65) and length increases, rendering the arteries tortuous; (2) both the wall intima (from 200 à 680 μm) and the media thicken and the arteries become rigid; (3) endothelial dysfunction is another major alteration associated with stiffness [95, 136]. The collagen content of the media increases with age, while the elastin content remains unchanged, which explains the increased arterial stiffness. Such a deregulation is a fairly complicated biological phenomenon since the increase of collagen protein is accompanied by a paradoxical reduction of the collagen messenger RNA and a paradoxical reduction of the collagenases [110, 111]. In addition, the collagen properties were altered by an age-specific process named glycation. Finally, the number of endothelial progenitors is reduced and this decrease has nothing to do with the increased arterial pressure [137].

One of the major components of arterial function in ageing is enhanced stiffness [105]. Arteries became less compliant and the aorta characteristic impedance, which is around 50 dyne·sec·cm^5 at 30 years, increases to 90 dyne·sec·cm^{-5} at 70 years. Such a rise results from the combination of different factors. Impedance is to pressure and pulsatile flow what resistance is to continuous flow. It expresses the relation between pressure and pulsatile flow registered at the same point on a vessel and, of course, depends on the peripheral resistance (impedance is enhanced in hypertension), but also on the inertance, compliance, diameter of the vessel, and the pulsatile wave back. These last three parameters are modified with age. Systolic arterial pressure increases while diastolic pressure is reduced, and pulse pressure is increased. Pulse pressure is the best marker of the vascular risk after 60; before this age, diastolic pressure is a better marker [95, 138–140].

The Micro-Vascular System
The microvascular endothelium is modified with ageing [141]. At present, these modifications are attributed to oxidative stress. They also include the lymphatic system and result in reduced capillary vasomotricity and capillary density, with a thickening of cerebral capillary walls and increased perivascular dermal hyaline deposits. In the brain, microcirculation may be hampered by the beta-amyloid substance 142].

6.5.3   Consequences of Change in Characteristic Arterial Impedance

The increase of impedance of the large arteries results in a left ventricular mechanical overload, without any modification of peripheral resistance. The LV and its cardiocytes are hypertrophied and this is accompanied by qualitative changes in species-specific myocardium composition discovered in our laboratory in 1979 [112, 143–145]. Modifications of pulmonary artery impedance have no real consequences for the right ventricle because, in the young, this impedance is extremely low. From a physiological point of view, the hypertrophy is compensated for. The contraction and relaxation of the heart of a 24- month-old rat (which is a senescent animal) is slowed, and the contractile cycle is thermodynamically more economic (see Glosssary) since the curvature of the Hill's relation is less pronounced [146, 147]. Another factor contributes to the formation of cardiac hypertrophy, the cellular losses, which may have an ischemic or an apoptotic origin [16].

The same alterations are found in the coronary arteries. They explain both the fall in coronary reserve and the increased sensitivity to ischemia, which are essential characteristics of the senescent heart and exist both in human beings and in mammals. Vascular tone, the endothelial function and the density of the coronary vascular bed are reduced with ageing. The coronary reserve is hampered and, in experimental data, for the same reduction of coronary flow, the senescent cardiac performances were more affected than those for the young. In addition, it has been shown by Patrick Assayag that the response to ischemia of the senescent coronary vessels is a vasoconstriction and not, like in the young vessels, a vasodilatation [101, 119].

6.5.4   The Clinical Manifestations of Atherosclerosis

Advanced atherosclerotic lesions are rich in SCs. Experimental models have evidenced the presence of a number of cytokines and chemokines in foam cells of atherosclerotic plaques, which are well-documented atherogenic inflammatory factors. In most advanced lesions like unstable plaques, the epithelial SCs participate in the instability by the secretome production of proteases that will degrade elastic fibers and thin the fibrous cover as well by the production of pro-inflammatory factors, which participate in the oxidation of the low-density lipoproteins, the LDLs [80, 148]. So, SCs are, at least on two different levels, essential components of the atherogenic process (Table 6.6).

The vascular endothelial SCs are also rich in miRs (miR143, miR145, miR126) that directly or indirectly possess atherogenic properties. Senescent arteries are

Table 6.6   The soluble and insoluble secretome of senescent endothelium in charge of atherosclerosis development. The major arguments

Senescent vascular smooth muscle cells, VSMC, are generally considered to contribute to atherosclerotic plaques by failure to proliferate, resulting in unstable fibrous cap. Gardner et al. [149] found that the secretome of human senescent VSMC, which is mainly located in the fibrous cap region, can promote chemotaxis of mononuclear cells both in vitro and in vivo by producing several cytokines (IL-6 and IL-8) and chemokines (such as the powerful chemoattractant protein 1, the macri = ophage inflammatory protein-1alpha, and many others), in an autocrine manner. The secretome also contains an active matrix metalloprotease and factors upregulating the inflammasome components and causing normal cells to release cytokins and upregulate adhesion molecules. Instead of being an inert component of the arterial wall, senescent VSMC actively participates in the atherosclerosis process.
The insoluble components of the SC secretome, i.e. the microvesicular miRs, also participate in atherogenesis. mir-143 and miR-145 prevent the dedifferentiation of the vascular cells; miR-126 activates the production of pro-inflammatoy factors [26] (see Table 4.3)

stiffer and longer than adult vessels and this is associated with a rise in systolic and pulse pressures, a well-documented risk factor.

In addition to this, age is associated with a longer exposure to various risk factors, arterial pressure, cholesterol, glycemia, excess calories, tobacco (active and passive), and pollution. The links with the CSs (above all endothelial) secretome are more complex, but, globally, "age linked inflammatory hyperstimulation favours inflammation within the atherosclerotic plaque." miRs represent an additional risk factor [26]. The relationships between atherosclerosis and inflammation are well-documented, and, for example, the senescent human vascular smooth cells secrete a variety of pathogenic compounds, including inflammatory factors and metalloproteases, all of which have atherogenic properties [7, 26, 27, 149–151].

6.5.5   Heart Failure in Senescence

Heart failure, HF, in old persons is frequent and, from a clinical point of view, not easily identified. As previously explained, ageing is associated with at least three diseases which can potentially modify the myocardial function, namely, atherosclerosis, arterial hypertension, and diabetes. In addition, the physiological performances of the senescent heart are reduced, while it is difficult, presently, to firmly establish a link between heart failure and the physiological characteristics of the senescent heart (see Sect. 6.5.1).

Heart failure with a preserved ejection fraction, HFpEF, is more commonly a disease of old persons [152]. The relationships between the senescent heart and HFpEF are still far from being fully elucidated despite the huge number of publications previously published on this topic [88, 153–159]. HFpEF is a heterogeneous clinical framework which, in the elderly, is as frequent as heart failure with reduced ejection fraction. This is truly a heterogeneous geriatric disease, associated with multiple cardiac (coronary insufficiency and atrial fibrillation) and noncardiac (diabetes, renal failure, frailty syndrome, and cognition dysfunctions) comorbidities. Several biomarkers of senescence are significantly associated with HFpEF, including telomere attrition and the elevation of certain miRs [152, 155, 160, 161].

Nevertheless, HFpEF has probably two specific features. (1) Fibrosis is present but modest [152]. (2) It is now possible, using speckle tracking, to explore the ventricular functioning by studying the ventricular torsion according to the scheme provided by Torrent-Guasp in 2001 [122, 124]. Age-linked torsion dysfunctioning was reported. The systolic torsion of the whole ventricle increases with ageing: the basal torsion is reduced while apical torsion increases, which strongly supports the hypothesis that anatomical abnormalities exist in the elderly [123, 162].

6.5.6   Atrial Fibrillation

Ageing is associated with the high prevalence of severe atrial fibrillation. Atrial remodeling concerns both the thickness and the size of atria, and, in addition, atrial tissue is more fibrotic. Atrial myocytes become hypertrophied and less numerous and interruptions in connection distribution hamper the propagation of electric waves. The result is a well-documented electrophysiological remodeling. Such remodeling is also associated with several other factors and comorbidities that favor the prevalence of atrial fibrillation in old persons [163]. It was recently suggested during the last congress of the American Heart Association (November 10–122018) that several biomarkers of senescence, like the tau protein or the Growth Differentiation Factor 15 level, were linked to the incidence of atrial fibrillation.

References

1. Callahan D, et al. The Quagmire. How American medicine is destroying itself. The New Republic 2011 May 19.
2. Foreman KJ, et al. Forecasting life expectancy years of life lost, and cause-specific mortality for 250 causes of death: reference and alternative scenarios for 2016-40 for 195 countries and territories. Lancet. 2018;392(10159):2052–90.
3. GBD 2016 Disease and Injury Incidence and Prevalence Collaborators. Global, regional, and national incidence, prevalence and years lived with disability for 328 diseases and injuries for 195 countries, 1990-2016: a systematic analysis for the GBDS 2016. Lancet. 2017;390:1211–59.
4. GBD 2016 DALYS and HALE Collaborators. Global, regional, and national disability-adjusted life-years (DALYS) for 333 diseases and injuries and healthy life expectancy (HALE) for 195 countries and territories, 1990-2016: a systematic analysis for the GBDS 2016. Lancet. 2017;390:1260–344.
5. Belmin J, et al., editors. Gériatrie. Paris: Elsevier/Masson; 2009. p. 835.
6. Naylor RM, et al. Senescent cells : a novel therapeutic target for aging and age-related diseases. Clin Pharmacol Ther. 2013;93:105–16.
7. Brondello JM, et al. La sénescence cellulaire.Un nouveau mythe de Janus? MédSci. 2012;28:288–94.
8. Rochefort H, et al. Endocrine disruptors (EDs) and hormone-dependent cancers: correlation or causal relationship? C R Biol. 2017;340:439–45.
9. Michaloglou C, et al. BRAF^{E600}-associated senescence-like cell cycle like arrest of human naevi. Nature. 2005;436:720–4.
10. Jonna S, et al. Geriatric assessment factors are associated with mortality after hospitalization in older adults with cancer. Support Care Cancer. 2016;24:4807–13.
11. Falandry C, et al. Biology of cancer and aging: a complex association with cellular senescence. J Clin Oncol. 2014;32:2604–10.
12. Finkel T, et al. The common biology of cancer and ageing. Nature. 2007;448:767–74.
13. Aunan JR, et al. The biology of aging and cancer: a brief overview of shared and divergent molecuar hallmarks. Aging Dis. 2017;8:628–42.
14. Tomasetti C, et al. Stem cell divisions, somatic mutations, cancer etiology, and cancer prevention. Science. 2017;355:1330–4.
15. Lakatta EG. So! What's aging? Is cardiovascular aging a disease? J Mol Cell Cardiol. 2015;83:1–13.
16. Swynghedauw B. Molecular mechanisms of myocardial remodeling. Physiol Rev. 1999;79:215–62.
17. Willis MS, et al. Proteotoxicity and cardiac dysfunction- Alzheimer's disease of the heart? N Engl J Med. 2013;368:454–64.
18. Floor SL, et al. Hallmarks of cancer: of all cancer cells all the time. Trends Mol Med. 2012;18:509.
19. Hanahan D, et al. Hallmarks of cancer: the next generation. Cell. 2011;144:647.
20. Hanahan D, et al. The hallmarks of cancer. Cell. 2000;100:57–70.
21. Jesus BB, et al. Telomerase at the intersection of cancer and aging. Trends Genet. 2013;29:513–20.
22. Stratton MR, et al. The cancer genome. Nature. 2009;458:719–24.

23. Hou L, et al. Blood telomere length attrition and cancer development in the normative aging study cohort. EBioMedicine. 2015;2:591–6.
24. Krtolica A, et al. Senescent fibroblasts promote epithelial cell growth and tumorigenesis: a link between cancer and aging. PNAS. 2001;98:12072–7.
25. Campisi J, et al. Aging, cellular senescence, and cancer. Annu Rev Physiol. 2013;75:685–705.
26. Weilner S, et al. Secretion of microvesicular miRNAs in cellular and organismal aging and age-related diseases. Exp Gerontol. 2013;48:626–33.
27. Camici GG, et al. Molecular mechanism of endothelial and vascular aging: implications for cardiovascular disease. Eur Heart J. 2015;36:3392–403.
28. Collado M, et al. Cellular senescence in cancer and aging. Cell. 2007;130:223–33.
29. Kennedy AL, et al. Activation of the PIK3CA/AKT pathway suppresses senescence induced by an activated RAS oncogene to promote tumorigenesis. Mol Cell. 2011;42:36–49.
30. Schultz MB, et al. When stem cells grow old: phenotype and mechanisms of stem cell aging. Development. 2018;143:3–14.
31. Davalos AR, et al. Senescent cells as a source of inflammatory factors for tumor progression. Cancer Metastasis Rev. 2010;29:273–83.
32. Jacob F. Evolution and tinkering. Science. 1977;196:1161–6.
33. Golde TE, et al. Proteinopathy-induced neuronal senescence: a hypothesis for brain failure in Alzheimer's and other neurodegenerative diseases. Alzheimer's Res Therap. 2009;1:5–17.
34. Weller RO, et al. Cerebrovascular disease is a major factor in the failure of elimination of Abeta from the aging human brain. Ann NY Acad Sci. 2002;977:162–8.
35. Jacqmin-Gadda H, et al. 20-year prevalence projections for dementia and impact of preventive policy about risk factors. Eur J Epidemiol. 2013;28:493–502.
36. Golde TE, et al. Thinking laterally about neurodegenerative proteinopathies. J Clin Invest. 2013;123:1847–55.
37. Weinstein G, et al. Risk estimations, risk factors, and genetic variants associated with Alzheimer's disease in selected publications from the Framingham heart study. J Alzheimers Dis. 2013;33:S439–45.
38. Glass DJ, et al. Some evolutionary perspectives on Alzheimer's disease pathogenesis and pathology. AlzheimersDement. 2012;8:343–51.
39. Selkoe DJ. Alzheimer's disease: genes, proteins, and therapy. Physiol Rev. 2001;81:741–66.
40. Venegas C, et al. Microglia-derived ASC specks cross-seed amyloid-beta in Alzheimer's disease. Nature. 2017;552:355–61.
41. Godet O, et al. Association of white-matter lesions with brain atrophy markers: the three-city Dijon MRI study. Cerebrovasc Dis. 2009;28:177–84.
42. Dubois B, et al. Research criteria fot the diagnosis of Alzheimer's disease: revising the NINCDS-ADRDA criteria. Lancet Neurol. 2007;6:734–46.
43. Hanon O, et al. Plasma amyloid levels within the Alzheimer's process and correlations with central biomarkers. Alzheimers Dement. 2018;14(7):858–68.
44. Levy-Noqueira M, et al. Alzheimer's disease diagnosis relies on a twofold clinical-biological algorithm: three memory clinic case report. J Alzheimers Dis. 2017;60:577–83.
45. Nakamura A, et al. High performance plasma amyloid-beta biomarkers for Alzheimer disease. Nature. 2018;554:249–54.
46. Bousiges O, Blanc F. Diagnostic values of cerebro-spinal fluid biomarkers in dementia with lewy bodies. Clin Chim Acta. 2019;490:222–8.
47. Bussian TJ, et al. Clearance of senescent glial cells prevents tau-dependent pathology and cognitive decline. Nature. 2018;562:578–82.
48. Scheff SW, et al. Is synaptic loss a unique hallmark of Alzheimer's diesase? Biochem Pharmacol. 2014;88:517–28.
49. de Wilde MC, et al. Meta-analysis of synaptic pathology in Alzheimer's disease reveals selective molecular vesicular machinery vulnerability. Alzheimers Dement. 2016;12:633–44.
50. Zhang Y, et al. Hypothalamic stem cells control ageing speed partly through exosomal miRNAs. Nature. 2017;548:52–7.
51. Fitzpatrick AWP, et al. Cryo-EM structures of tau filaments from Alzheimer's disease. Nature. 2017;547:185–90.
52. Alvergne A, et al. Evolutionary thinking in medicine. Berlin: Springer; 2015.

53. Taylor RC, et al. Aging as an event of proteostasis collapse. Cold Spring Harb Perspect Biol. 2011;3:a004440.
54. Golde TE, et al. Proteinopathy-induced neuronal senescence: a hypothesis for brain failure in Alzheimer's and other neurodegenerative diseases. Alzheimers Res Ther. 2009;1:5–17.
55. Bhat R, et al. Astrocyte senescence as a component of Alzheimer's disease. PLoS ONE. 2012;7:e45069.
56. Bellingham SA, et al. Exosomes: vehicles for the transfer of toxic proteins associated with neurodegenerative diseases. Front Physiol. 2012;3:124.
57. Leidinger P, et al. A blood-based 12-miRNA signature of Alzheimer disease patients. Genome Biol. 2013;14:R78.
58. Ransohoff RM. How neuro-inflammation contributes to neuro-degeneration. Science. 2016;353:777–84.
59. Vermeij WP, et al. Restricted diet delays accelerated ageing and genomic stress in DNA-repair-deficient mice. Nature. 2016;532:427–31.
60. Jucker M, Walker LC. Self-propagation of pathogenic protein aggregates in neurodegenerative diseases. Nature. 2013;501:45–51.
61. Itzhaki RF, et al. Microbes and Alzheiner's disease. J Alzheimers Dis. 2016;51:979–84.
62. Abbott A. The red-hot debate about transmissible Alzheimer's. Nature. 2016;531:294–7.
63. Leon LJ, et al. Staying young at heat: autophagy and adaptation to cardiac aging. J Mol Cell Cardiol. 2016;95:78–85.
64. Fox M, et al. Hygiene and the world distribution of Alzhzeimer's disease. Evol Med Public Health. 2013;2013:173–86.
65. Elbaz A, et al. Professional exposure to pesticides and Parkinson disease. Ann Neurol. 2009;66:494–504.
66. Marano F, et al. Toxique ? Santé et environnement: de l'alerte la décision. Paris: Buchet-Chastel; 2015.
67. MacDade E, et al. Stop Alzheimer's before it starts. Nature. 2017;547:153–5.
68. Bredesen DE. Reversal of cognitive decline: a novel therapeutic program. Aging. 2014;6:707–17.
69. Aisen PS, et al. What we have learned from Expedition III and EPOCH trials? Perspective of the CTAD task force. J Prev Alzheimers Dis. 2018;5:171–4.
70. Fuchsberger C, et al. The genetic architecture of type 2 diabetes. Nature. 2016;536:41–7.
71. Chia CW, et al. Age-related changes in glucose metabolism, hyperglycemia, and cardiovascular risk. Circ Res. 2018;123:886–904.
72. Lee PG, et al. The pathophysiology of hyperglycemia in older adults: clinical considerations. Diabetes Care. 2017;40:444–52.
73. Poitout V, et al. Minireview: secondary beta-cell failure in type 2 diabetes: a convergence of glucotoxicity and lipotoxicity. Endocrinology. 2002;143:339–42.
74. Swynghedauw B, et al. Effects of IV injection of glucose on blood triglycerides in normal and diabetic subjects. Rev Fr Etudes Clin Biol. 1965;10(4):427–30.
75. Einstein FH, et al. Enhanced activation of a "nutrient sensing" pathways with age contributes to insulin-resistance. FASEB J. 2008;22:3450–7.
76. Dirks AJ, et al. Mitochondrial DNA mutations, energy metabolism and apoptosis in aging muscle. Ageing Res Rev. 2006;5:179–96.
77. Barzilai N, et al. The critical role of metabolic pathways in aging. Diabetes. 2012;61:1315–22.
78. Sone H, et al. Pancreatic beat cell senescence contributes to the pathogenesis of type 2 diabetes in high-fat diet-induced diabetic mice. Diabetologia. 2005;48:58–67.
79. Hotamisligil GS. Inflammation, metaflammation and immunometabolic disorders. Nature. 2017;542:177–85.
80. Childs BG, et al. Senescent intimal foam cells are deleterious at all stages of atherosclerosis. Science. 2016;354:472–7.
81. Bartling B. Cellular senescence in normal and premature lung aging. Z Gerontol Geriatr. 2013;46:613–22.
82. Chilosi M, et al. The pathogenesis of COPD and IPF: distinct horns for the same devil? Respir Res. 2012;13:3.

83. Hashimoto M, et al. Elimination of p19ARF-expressing cells enhances pulmonary function in mice. JCI Insight. 2016;1:e87732.
84. Schafer MJ, et al. Cellular senescence mediates fibrotic pulmonary disease. Nat Commun. 2017;8:1–11.
85. Sturmlechner I, et al. Cellular senescence in renal ageing and disease. Nat Rev Nephrol. 2017;13:77–89.
86. Schmitt R, Melk A. Molecular mechanisms of renal aging. Kidney Int. 2017;92(3):569–79.
87. Krizhanovsky V, et al. Senescence of activated stellate cells limits fibrosis. Cell. 2008;134:657–67.
88. Lakatta EG, et al. Perspectives on mammalian cardiovascular aging: human to molecules. Comp Biochem Physiol A Mol Integr Physiol. 2002;132:699–721.
89. Lakatta EG, Levy D. Arterial and cardiac aging: major shareholders in cardiovascular disease enterprises. Part I: aging arteries: a "set up" for vascular disease. Circulation. 2003;107:139–46.
90. Lakatta EG, Levy D. Arterial and cardiac aging: major shareholders in cardiovascular disease enterprises. Part II: the aging heart in health: links to heart disease. Circulation. 2003;107:346–54.
91. Lakatta EG, Levy D. Arterial and cardiac aging: major shareholders in cardiovascular disease enterprises. Part III: cellular and molecular clues to heart and arterial aging. Circulation. 2003;107:490–7.
92. Rozenberg S, et al. Severe impairment of ventricular compliance accounts for advanced age-associated hemodynamic dysfunction in rats. Exp Gerontol. 2006;41:289–95.
93. Swynghedauw B, editor. Hypertrophy and heart failure. Paris Londres: INSERM/J. LIBBEY pub; 1990.
94. Swynghedauw B. Les racines dixneuviémistes de la révolution biologique contemporaine. Hist Sci Med. 2006;40:141–50.
95. Levy B, et al. Biology of the arterial wall. Boston: Kluwer Academic Pub; 1999.
96. Burton DGA, et al. Pathophysiology of vascular calcification: pivotal role of cellular senescence in vascular smooth cells. Exp Gerontol. 2010;45:819–24.
97. Ieda M, et al. Cardiac fibroblasts regulate myocardial proliferation through beta 1 integrin signaling. Dev Cell. 2009;16:233–44.
98. Raggi P, et al. Coronary artery calcium to predict mortality in elderly men and women. J Am Coll Cardiol. 2008;52:17–23.
99. Anderson R, et al. Mechanisms driving the ageing heart. Exp Gerontol. 2018;109:5–15.
100. Rodeheffer RJ, et al. Exercise cardiac output is maintained with advancing age in healthy human subjects: cardiac dilatation and increased stroke volume compensate for diminished heart rate. Circulation. 1984;69:203–13.
101. Assayag P, et al. Effects of low-flow ischemia on myocardial function and calcium-regulating proteins in adult and senescent rat hearts. Cardiovasc Res. 1998;38:169–80.
102. Boluyt MO, et al. Echocardiographic assessment of age-associated changes in systolic and diastolic function of the female F344 rat heart. J Appl Physiol. 2004;96:822–8.
103. Pacher P, et al. Left ventricular pressure-volume relationship in a rat model of advanced aging-associated heart failure. Am J Phys. 2004;287:H2132–7.
104. Bergmann O, et al. Evidence for cardiomyocyte renewal in adults. Science. 2009;324:98–102.
105. Corman B, et al. Aminoguanidine prevents age-related arterial stiffening and cardiac hypertrophy. Proc Natl Acad Sci U S A. 1998;95:1301–6.
106. Gude NA, et al. Cardiac ageing: extrinsic and intrinsic factors in cellular renewal and senescence. Nat Rev Cardiol. 2018;15:523–42.
107. Kajstura J, et al. Cardiomyogenesis in the aging and failing human heart. Circulation. 2012;126:1869–81.
108. Malliaras K, et al. Cardiomyocyte proliferation and progenitor cell recruitment underlie therapeutic regeneration after myocardial infarction in the adult mouse heart. EMBO Mol Med. 2013;5:191–209.
109. Senyo SE, et al. Cardiac regeneration based on mechanisms of cardiomyocyte proliferation and differentiation. Stem Cell Res. 2014;13:532–41.

110. Besse S, et al. Nonsynchronous changes in myocardial collagen mRNA and protein during aging: effect of Doca-salt hypertension. Am J Phys. 1994;267:H2237–44.
111. Besse S, et al. Is the senescent heart overloaded and already failing ?A review. Cardiovasc Drug Ther (Invit Editor). 1994;8:581–7.
112. Lompré AM, et al. Myosin isoenzyme redistribution in chronic heart overloading. Nature. 1979;282:105–7.
113. Benetos A, et al. Short telomeres are associated with increased carotid atherosclerosis in hypertensive subjects. Hypertension. 2004;43:182–5.
114. Calado RT, Young NS. Telomere diseases. N Engl J Med. 2009;361:2353–65.
115. Benetos A, et al. Short leukocyte telomere length precedes clinical expression of atherosclerosis. The blood-and-muscle model. Circ Res. 2018;122:616–23.
116. Swynghedauw B, et al. Le pourquoi du vieillissement. In: Artigou JY, et al., editors. Traité de cardiologie.SFC. Paris: Elsevier Masson; 2007. p. 1201–3.
117. Swynghedauw B. Phenotypic plasticity of adult myocardium: molecular mechanisms. J Exp Biol. 2009;209(Pt 12):2320–7.
118. Swynghedauw B. Developmental and functional adaptation of contractile proteins in cardiac and skeletal muscle. Physiol Rev. 1986;66:710–71.
119. Assayag P, et al. Senescent heart as compared to pressure overload induced hypertrophy. Hypertension. 1997;29:15–21.
120. Weber KT. Wound healing in cardiovascular disease. Armonk: Futura Publishing Cy; 1995.
121. Weber KT, et al. Myofibroblast-mediated mechanisms of pathological remodelling of the heart. Nat Rev Cardiol. 2013;10:15–26.
122. Buckberg GD, et al. Left ventricular form and function.Scientific priorities and strategic planning for development of new views of the disease. Circulation. 2004;110:e333–6.
123. Hung C-L, et al. Age- and sex-related influences on left ventricular mechanics in elderly individuals free of prevalent heart failure. The ARIC Study (atherosclerosis risk in communities). Circ Cardiovasc Imaging. 2017;10:e004510.
124. Torrent-Guasp F, et al. The structure and function of the helical heart and its buttress wrapping. I. The normal macroscopic structure of the heart. Semin Thorac Cardiovasc Surg. 2001;13:301–19.
125. McLendon PM, Robbins J. Proteotoxicity and cardiac disfunction. Circ Res. 2015;116:1863–82.
126. Nakayama H, et al. Macromolecular degradation systems and cardiovascular aging. Circ Res. 2016;118:1577–92.
127. Henning RH, et al. Proteostasis in cardiac health and disease. Nat Rev Cardiol. 2017;14:637–53.
128. Mizushima W, et al. BAG3 plays a central role in proteostasis in the heart. J Clin Invest. 2017;127:2900–3.
129. Blice-Baum AC, et al. Modest overexpression of FOXO maintains cardiac proteostasis and ameliorate age-associated functional decline. Aging Cell. 2017;16:93–103.
130. Sanbe A, et al. Desmin-related cardiomyopathy in transgenic mice.: a cardiac amyloidosis. Proc Natl Acad Sci U S A. 2004;101:10132–6.
131. Logeart D, et al. Evidence of cardiac myolysis in severe nonischemic heart failure and the potential role of increased wall strain. Am Heart J. 2001;141:247–53.
132. Kostin S, et al. Myocytes die by multiple mechanisms in failing human hearts. Circ Res. 2003;92:715–24.
133. Baker DJ, et al. Clearance of p16[Ink4a]-positive cells delays ageing-associated disorders. Nature. 2011;479:232–6.
134. Barral JM, et al. Role of the myosin assembly protein UNC-45 as a molecular chaperone for myosin. Science. 2002;295:665–71.
135. Tanskanen M, et al. Senile systemic amyloidosis affects 25% of the very aged and associates with genetic variation in alpha2-macroglobulin and tau: a population-based autopsy study. Ann Med. 2009;40:232–9.
136. Donato AJ, et al. Mechanisms of dysfunction in the aging vasculature and the role in age-related disease. Circ Res. 2018;123:825–48.

137. Umemura T, et al. Aging and hypertension are independent risk factors for reduced number of circulating endothelial progenitor cells. Am J Hypertens. 2008;21:1203–9.
138. Plouin PF, et al. L'hypertension artérielle du sujet âgé. Bull Acad Natl Méd. 2006;190:793–806.
139. Safar M. Ageing and its effects on the cardiovascular system. Drugs. 1990;39(suppl I):1–8.
140. Minamino T, et al. Vascular senescence and vascular aging. J Mol Cell Cardiol. 2004;36:175–83.
141. Levy B, et al., editors. Role of the micro and macrocirculation in target organ damage in diabetes and hypertension. Hoboken: Wiley; 2009.
142. Scioli MG, et al. Ageing and microvasculature. Vasc Cell. 2014;6:19.
143. Klotz C, et al. Evidence for new forms of cardiac myosin heavy chains in mechanical heart overloading and in ageing. Eur J Biochem. 1981;115:415–21.
144. Mercadier JJ, et al. Myosin heavy chain and atrial size in patients with various types of mitral valve dysfunction: a quantitative study. J Am Coll Cardiol. 1987;9:1024–30.
145. Swynghedauw B, et al. Species-specificity of the isomyosin shift in cardiac overload. J Appl Cardiol. 1988;3:133–43.
146. Boutouyrie P, et al. Common carotid artery stiffness patterns of left ventricular hypertrophy in hypertensive patients. Hypertension. 1995;25:651–9.
147. Staessen JA, et al. Essential hypertension. Lancet. 2003;361:1629–41.
148. Minamino T, et al. Endothelial senescence in human atherosclerosis: role oftelomer in endothelial dysfunction. Circulation. 2002;105:1541–4.
149. Gardner SE, et al. Senescent vascular smooth muscle cells drive inflammation through an interleukin-1alpha dependent senescent-associated secretory phenotype. Arterioscler Thromb Vasc Biol. 2015;35:1963–074.
150. Boddaert J, et al. Ch. 20 L'athérosclérose et ses interactions avec le vieillissement. In: Assayag P, et al., editors. Traité de médecine CV du sujet âge. Paris: Flammarion; 2007.
151. Rodier F, Campisi J. Four faces of cellular senescence. J Cell Biol. 2011;192:547–56.
152. Upadhya B, et al. Evolution of a geriatric syndrome: pathophysiology and treatment of heart failure with preserved ejection function. J Am Ger Soc. 2017;65:2431–40.
153. De Keulenaer GW, et al. Are systolic and diastolic heart failure overlapping or distinct phenotypes within the heart failure spectrum? Circulation. 2011;123:1996–2005.
154. Lewis GA, et al. Biological phenotypes of heart failure with preserved ejection fraction. J Am Coll Cardiol. 2017;70:2186–200.
155. Loffredo FS, et al. Heart failure with preserved ejection fraction: molecular pathways of the aged myocardium. Circ Res. 2014;115:97–107.
156. Owan TE, et al. Trends in prevalence and outcome of heart failure with preserved ejection fraction. N Engl J Med. 2006;355:251–9.
157. Shah AM, et al. Contemporary assessment of left ventricular diastolic function in older adults. The atherosclerosis risk in communities study. Circulation. 2017;135:426–39.
158. Shah SJ, et al. Phenomapping for novel classification of heart failure with preserved ejection function. Circulation. 2015;131:269–79.
159. Sharma K, et al. Heart failure with preserved ejection function: mechanisms, clinical features, and therapies. Circ Res. 2014;115:79–96.
160. Boon RA, et al. MicroRNA-34a regulates cardiac ageing and function. Nature. 2013;495:107–10.
161. Borlaug BA, et al. Heart failure with preserved ejection fraction: pathophysiology, diagnosis, and treatment. Eur Heart J. 2011;32:670–9.
162. Kaku K, et al. Age-related normal range of left ventricular strain and torsion using three-dimensional speckle-tracking echocardioagraphy. J Am Soc Echocardiogr. 2014;27:55–64.
163. Lin YK, et al. Aging modulates the substrate and triggers remodeling in atrial fibrillation. Circ J. 2018;82(5):1237–44.

How to Treat or Prevent, or Slow Down, Cellular Ageing and Senescence?

7

Abstract

For the moment, calorie restrictions and exercising are the only validated therapies for treating or slowing ageing. Various attempts at reprogramming, based on the cellular senescence concept, have been developed, but, for the moment, without any clinical applications.

The fact that life span and health span have not increased at the same pace is a major concern. Treating or preventing ageing is an old problem and for the moment calorie restriction and exercising are the only validated therapies.

For those who are in charge of health-care systems, the prevention of unhealthy ageing is a major public problem [1, 2]. Calorie restriction and exercising are, for the moment, the unique "treatments" of senescence, which have been fully and reproducibly validated, in humans. Both act, at least in part, through a reduction of inflammatory factors. The subject is of major importance from both a health and an economic point of view. Hundreds of other therapies have been tried, but with no success at present.

7.1 The Various Attempts at Reprogramming

Many experiments or trials based on the concept previously developed have been initiated and carried out in order to prevent or slow down the senescent process. These "senotherapies" mostly target SCs [3–5] (Table 7.1).

An important progress in developing anti-ageing drugs was the development of a senescence-associated beta-galactosidase assay as a screening platform to rapidly identify drugs that could potentially have senolytic properties. Ercc1$^{-/-}$ murine fibroblasts with reduced DNA repair capacities and which senesce rapidly when grown in atmospheric oxygen have been successfully tried [6]. The authors cover a

Table 7.1 The senescent cell, the real target for prevention and therapy

The mechanisms that drive ageing might also promote age-related diseases. Cellular senescence is a permanent state of cell cycle arrest, which has recently emerged as a fundamental ageing mechanism and also contributes to diseases of late life, including cancer, atherosclerosis, and osteoarthritis. Safe therapeutic strategies would include selective elimination of SCs or disruption of their secretome. They are now nearing human trials

fairly unlimited number of diets or food approaches, as well as several biological or chemical compounds such as sirtuins [7], rapamycin, inhibitors of the HSPs (e.g., 17-DMAG, an inhibitor of HSP 90, see [6]), spermidine, metformin [8, 9], hydrogen sulfide, several compounds of the secretome, even the microbiota, and compounds altering the autophagy process [10]. For the moment none of these trials have provided convincing evidence for their efficacy and reproducibility (see the critical review of [1, 11] and the site *COST Action BM 1402* from the European Community). Following the work of Baker [12, 13], several trials have been conducted so far on experimental models in order to increase life span and reduce the frequency of age-linked diseases by suppressing SCs. A good example is the work of Baar [14] who was using various activators of apoptosis. Such strategies include trials aimed at comorbidities and various age-linked diseases, which are associated with the excess of SCs [2]. Innovative strategies based on the well-documented plasticity of both resident stem cells and differentiated cells [15], such as spurring senescent stem cells, are still in development.

Another potential tool were data from JM Lemaitre's group, showing the possibility of a direct reprogramming of human centenarians pluripotent SCs. These reprogrammed SCs were indistinguishable from induced pluripotent stem cells from young persons and is an important step toward regenerative medicine in aged persons [16].

Many experiments using parabiosis were carried out in animals by cross-linking the circulations of young and old animals. The interpretation of these results is not always easy; nevertheless, for the moment, the papers published using this technology showed that young blood may improve the performances of old animals and that, conversely, blood from old animals worsened the health conditions of younger animals. Interestingly, the inhibitory effects of old blood were more pronounced than the benefits of young blood. Such results are highly suggestive of a determinant role of components of the SC secretome [17].

Epigenetic modifications can be reversed in some models. This was the origin of several designs planned for new anti-ageing treatments, like administration of histone deacetylase inhibitor in progeroid mice to extend their life span and reduce the incidence of brain disease [18].

During development, cell differentiation is far from perfect. With time, the mechanisms that protect the cell against degradation become less and less efficient and cellular deterioration accumulates. Cellular homeostasis (e.g., proteostasis see Sect. 3.4 and accompanying figures) is finally compromised [18]. Nevertheless, it was recently shown in a mouse model of premature ageing (progeria) that partial cellular reprogramming to pluripotency by forced short-term cyclic expression of the so-called "Yamanaka factors" in charge of the global remodeling of epigenetic marks improves several hallmarks of ageing. Such genome remodeling modifies the expression of several genes associated with epigenetic dysregulation and results in increased resistance to metabolic disease, without the emergence of tumors [19].

7.2   Calorie Restriction

The enhancement of life span by calorie restriction is extremely well-documented in many experimental models (from flies, such as Drosophila, to mice including also nematodes) [20, 21, 36], as also in humans, although two studies in Primates provided some contradictory results (see [1]). A sociohistorical turn in 2006, when the number of deaths caused by obesity exceeded those linked to starvation [1] (Table 7.2). Calorie restriction has positive effects not only on the incidence of CV diseases, but also on verbal memory, probability of age-related dementia, and bouts of depression. These positive effects utilize a common metabolic pathway (insulin/insulin-like growth factor 1 signaling/TOR pathway), which is central and also well-conserved throughout evolution history [20]. The pathway can be inhibited

Table 7.2 Caloric restriction to treat or prevent senescence

Calorie restriction, CR, and energy homeostat for Speakman et al. [23]
Experimentally, calorie restriction has several beneficial effects; it prevents cancer, CV and neurodegenerative diseases and enhances life span. This has been extremely well-documented for more than 100 years. Studies in humans are still limited but are highly suggestive that CR may have similar benefits in humans. The constant hunger, reduced thermoregulation, and loss of libido makes CR unattractive for human beings and has induced the development of several drugs, also called CR mimetic drugs—such as resveratrol, rapamycin or metformin, to mimic the metabolic effects of CR. "Ultimately, then, the main problem with CR mimetics may not be their development, but the wholescale restructuring of the medical and drug establishment to permit their use." The problem is likely to be far from exclusive biological considerations and belongs more to health organization

The anti-ageing effects of CR for Cintron-Colon et al. [24]
In endothermic animals, CR lowers core body temperature, as a component of the adaptive mechanism to conserve energy until food becomes available. The authors found, in the mouse, that the insulin-like growth factor controls this response and that regulation was carried out by the central nervous system. During CR, the genetic or pharmacological (dose-dependent) inhibition of IGF-1R enhanced the reduction of both core body temperature and energy expenditure. Targeted, central but not peripheral, knockout of the signal selectively in forebrain neuron reveals that this regulation was located in the regions rostral of the canonical hypothalamic nuclei. For example, after ubiquitous ablation of IGF-1R, the hypothermic response to 50% CR was more pronounced than in controls. CR, IGF-1R signaling and body temperature that regulates metabolism, ageing, and longevity are in fact components of the same pathways
Several HSP90 inhibitors or autophagy regulators were selected, such as 17 DMAG, quercetin or navitoclax, using this screening platform; nevertheless, for the moment, although these components have senolytic activity in vitro and also in vivo in mice, the general thinking is that they will probably be more effective in association with other drugs that target, for example, the apoptotic pathway

with positive consequences on the average life span by using either mutagenesis or several drugs such as rapamycin [21] or metformin [8]. Calorie restriction is also known to induce a correct "rewiring" of the circadian rhythm, which is strongly modified in senescence [25].

7.3   Physical Exercise

The beneficial effects of physical exercise are also extremely well-documented (Table 7.3) [27]; they are even going to be refunded by the Social security system, at least in France. Muscular activity activates the autocrine production of a secretome [28, 29]. These data complete the already published findings involving another transcription cofactor, PGC 1alpha. This cofactor has a pleiotropic activity, which accounts for the well-documented effects of exercise on the expression of several metabolic genes, and also on the genes involved in muscle protein synthesis, angiogenesis, inflammation, and oxidation ([26, 30–36]; see above all [37, 38]).

Experiments, as well as clinical trials, have evidenced an exercise-induced activation of telomerase and of several factors controlling its activity (Table B1 and Fig. 7.1) [37, 38]. Telomere length starts to be reduced after 50 years and physical exercise facilitates a full recovery of their length during youth. Exercise activates the expression of genes encoding proteins that stabilize the telomere both in mice and in human beings, both in the leukocytes and in the aortic wall. The underlying mechanism involves an activation of eNOS and a synergic activation of the telomerase and several markers of senescence, which are protectors against apoptosis. Importantly, telomerase activation not only controls telomere length but has broader effects. TFR2, a factor that regulates telomerase activity is activated by physical

Table 7.3 Health benefits of physical activity (from [26])

	Level of evidence (*dose/response*)
– All causes global mortality (regular physical activity >2000 kcal/ week, increases life span at 80 years by 2 years)	+++ (*yes*)
CV diseases	
– Primary prevention (mortality, sudden death, hypertension)	+++ (review) (*yes*)
– Secondary prevention (coronary insufficiency and heart failure)	+++ (meta-analysis)
Type 2 diabetes	
– Primary prevention	+++ (review) (*yes*)
– Secondary prevention	+++ (meta-analysis)
Cancer	
– Primary prevention: breast, colon	+++ (*yes*)
– Secondary prevention	+
Post-menopausal osteoporosis	
– Primary prevention (fractures, bone density)	++ (big series)
– Secondary prevention Primary prevention	(*possible*) + (preliminary)
General condition	
– Well-being, quality of life, psychological state	+++ (two reviews)

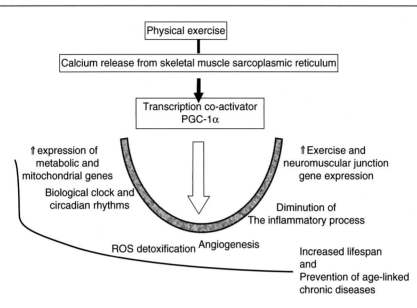

Fig. 7.1 Exercise increases life span, but how does it operate? Calcium release during exercise activates a strong multipotent coactivator of transcription. This coactivator can itself activate in a coordinated fashion the transcription of several groups of homogeneous genes that, in turn, may either activate the protein synthesis of the muscle mass and its vessels or inhibit the inflammatory process. PGC-1 alpha: coactivator-1 alpha of the Peroxisome-Proliferator-Activated Receptor-gamma. ROS: reactive oxygen species

exercise and is involved independently in both the regulation of telomere length and the regulation of the senescent process. Exercise inhibits several regulators of the cell cycle and this inhibition disappears if telomerase activity is suppressed by transgenic manipulations.

References

1. de Cabo R, et al. The search for antiaging interventions: from elixirs to fasting regimens. Cell. 2014;157:1515–26.
2. Kirkland JL, et al. The clinical potential of senolytic drugs. J Am Geriatr Soc. 2017;65:2297–301.
3. van Deursen JM. The role of senescent cells in ageing. Nature. 2014;509:439–46.
4. Schmitt R. Senotherapy: growing old and staying young ? Pflugers Arch. 2017;469:1051–9.
5. Childs BG, et al. Senescent cells: an emerging target for diseases of ageing. Nat Rev Drug Discov. 2017;16:718–35.
6. Fuhrmann-Strissnigg H, et al. Identification of HS90 inhibitors as a novel class of senolytics. Nat Commun. 2017;8:422.
7. Kane AE, et al. Sirtuins and NAD+ in the development and treatment of metabolic and cardio-vascular diseases. Circ Res. 2018;123:868–85.
8. Gallagher EJ, et al. Diabetes, cancer, and metformin: connections of metabolism and cell pro-liferation. Ann N Y Acad Sci. 2011;1243:54–68.
9. Noren Hooten N, et al. Metformin-mediated increase in DICR1 regulates microRNA expres-sion and cellular senescence. Aging Cell. 2016;15:572–81.

10. Abdellatif M, et al. Autophagy in cardiovascular aging. Circ Res. 2018;123:803–24.

11. Bellantuono I, et al. Find drugs that delay many diseases of old age. Nature. 2018;554:293–5.

12. Baker DJ, et al. Clearance of p16^{Ink4a}-positive cells delays ageing-associated disorders. Nature. 2011;479:232–6.

13. Baker DJ, et al. Naturally occurring p16^{Ink4a}-positive cells shorten healthy lifespan. Nature. 2016;530:184–9.

14. Baar MP, et al. Targeted apoptosis of senescent cells restores tissue homeostasis in response to chemotoxicity and ageing. Cell. 2017;169:132–47.

15. Wells JM, et al. Diverse mechanisms for endogenous regeneration and repair in mammalian organs. Nature. 2018;557:322–8.

16. Lapasset L, et al. Rejuvenating senescent and centenarian human cells by reprogramming through the pluripotent state. Genes Dev. 2011;25:2248–53.

17. Rebo J, et al. A single heterochronic blood exchange reveals rapid inhibition of multiple tissue by old blood. Nat Commun. 2016;7:13363. https://doi.org/10.1038/ncomms13363.

18. Lopez-Otin C, et al. The hallmarks of ageing. Cell. 2013;153:1194.

19. Ocampo A, et al. Amelioration of age-associated hallmark by partial reprogramming. Cell. 2016;167:1719–33.

20. Fontana L, et al. Dietary restriction, growth factors and ageing: form yeast to humans. Science. 2010;328:321–6.

21. Gems D, et al. Genetics of longevity in models organisms: debates and paradigms shifts. Annu Rev Physiol. 2013;75:621–44.

22. Chung HY, et al. Molecular inflammation: underpinnings of ageing and age-related diseases. Ageing Res Rev. 2009;8:18–30.

23. Speakman JR, et al. Caloric restriction. Mol Asp Med. 2011;32:159–221.

24. Cintron-Colon R, et al. Insulin-like growth factor 1 receptor regulates hypothermia during calorie restriction. Proc Natl Acad Sci U S A. 2017;114:9731–6.

25. Touitou Y, et al. Modifications of circadian and circannual rhythms with ageing. Exp Gerontol. 1997;32:603–14.

26. Swynghedauw B. L'exercice physique, seul traitement validé du vieillissement. Evidence. Limites. Mécanismes. Revue de gériatrie. Mars 2009.

27. Warburton DER, et al. Health benefits of physical activity: a systematic review of current systematic reviews. Curr Opin Cardiol. 2017;32:541–56.

28. Bouzki K, et al. Bimodal effect on pancreatic beat cells of secretory products from normal or insulin-resistant human skeletal muscle. Diabetes. 2011;60:1111–21.

29. Hojman P, et al. Exercise-induced muscle-derived cytokines inhibit mammary cancer cell growth. Am J Physiol Endocrinol Metab. 2011;301:E504–10.

30. Benetos A, et al. Short telomeres are associated with increased carotid atherosclerosis in hypertensive subjects. Hypertension. 2004;43:182–5.

31. Calado RT, Young NS. Telomere diseases. N Engl J Med. 2009;361:2353–65.

32. Fleg JL. Exercise therapy for older heart failure patients. Heart Fail Clin. 2017;13:607–17.

33. Kasch FW, et al. Ageing of the cardiovascular system during 33 years of aerobic exercise. Age Ageing. 1999;28:531–6.

34. Pedersen BK, et al. Muscles, exercise and obesity: skeletal muscle as a secretory organ. Nat Rev Endocrinol. 2012;8:457–65.

35. Werner C, et al. Physical exercise prevents cellular senescence in circulating leukocytes and in the vessel wall. Circulation. 2009;120:2438–47.

36. Vermeij WP, et al. Restricted diet delays accelerated ageing and genomic stress in DNA-repair-deficient mice. Nature. 2016;532:427–31.

37. Finck BN, Kelly DP. PGC-1 coactivators: inducible regulators of energy metabolism in health and disease. J Clin Invest. 2006;116:615–22.

38. Handschin C, et al. The role of exercise and PGC-1a in inflammation and chronic disease. Nature. 2008;454:463–9.

Senescence: A Darwinian Evolutionary Perspective

8

Abstract

Senescence is a property of every living species and is linked to the evolutionary law formulated by Darwin. Nevertheless, "senescence" still requires a general definition covering the three phylogenetic kingdoms of life. In mammalians, senescence is linked to inflammation.

Senescence is a property of every living species, including bacteria and plants. The contemporary increase in mean life span results entirely from human activity, including improvements in hygiene, progress in medicine or improvement in life-style, comfort, food supply, etc. [1], this is why we can say with Oscar Burger [2] that in 2017, ageing, ageing well, is contrary to biological evolution. The same is true for other species which live in our proximity as pets and are highly dependent on human activity.

Charles Darwin [3] summarized his evolutionary theory with the following shortcut, "descent with modifications." Evolution proceeds by selective pressure and aims to improve the reproductive capacity, the so-called Darwinian fitness (Fig. 8.1). A mutation occurring by chance can provide the bearer with an advantage, and because of this advantage, is stored; conversely, deleterious or useless mutations will progressively disappear. This rationale implies that the bearer of the mutation is young enough to be able to transmit the mutation to a progeny. Evolution gave rise to a new field, evolutionary medicine initiated in 1995 by an American psychiatrist, Randolph Nesse [4]. See also Trevathan [5], Flatt [6], Phelan [7], and many others [8]. In French, see Swynghedauw [9] and Frelin [10].

© Springer Nature Switzerland AG 2019

B. Swynghedauw, *The Biology of Senescence*, Practical Issues in Geriatrics,

https://doi.org/10.1007/978-3-030-15111-9_8

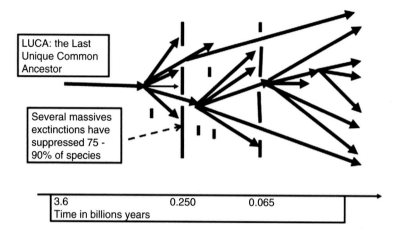

Fig. 8.1 The phylogenetic evolutionary tree. Evolution signifies that every living species has a common ancestor (called LUCA, for last unique common ancestor). Evolution proceeds as an evolutionary tree by chance and necessity, chance providing different gamete rearrangements and necessity selecting the ones which are the most useful for reproduction. There are also catastrophies that eliminate most living species. Two of them are documented in the past, the last suppressed 90% of species, including dinosaurs

8.1   Genetic Versus Environmental Factors in Senescence

The complicated relationships between our genetic individual background and our collectively acquired environmental factors reflect the complexity of life, and it is not surprising that such complexity is equally observed during ageing. Ageing is not driven by genetic programming towards death [11]. The progressive deterioration of physiological function is by no means universal. There are living species in which senescence is modular such as plants [12], salmon age once, they die just after reproducing.

Genetic, hereditary factors are the first factors responsible for the maximum life span of a given living species and the maximum life span is clearly a full characteristic of a species which signifies that during evolution in human species like in every other living species, the genome was shaped so as to delineate its maximum life span. For us, it is a little more than a hundred years. This is our own living species characteristic [13].

A recent detailed study by Jones [14] concerning 40 different living species belonging to different families (mammalians, or other vertebrates, "invertebrates" vascular plants, algae) evidenced the extreme diversity of the maximum life span and of the fertility periods, from one species to another (a dozen minutes in some bacteria, a few days in certain plants, up to a hundred years in sequoia or sharks).

Our genome mirrors how everyone copes with his own environment. It is between these limits that life span is defined, based on the environmental data (climate, standard of life, access to therapies, etc.) presented to us. The Darwinian "evolutionary theory" is no longer a theory, but a biological law, an evolutionary basis of biology, and is now supported by thousands of papers. This evolutionary basis of ageing "cannot be described as a genetically programmed phenomenon on a par with development" [15].

The most simple theory of ageing is that which supposes that ageing is caused by the accumulation over time of various mutations or gene defects. This notion of accumulation is no longer questionable [16], but it does not explain the recent evolution of mean life span in good health [2], even if we add that the DNA repair processes, it may be attenuated with ageing.

The antagonistic theory postulates that the genes driving ageing have been selected because they provide an advantage early in life despite their deleterious effects in elders. The elderly may express genes whose penetrance is delayed, as for the Huntington's chorea gene that is expressed late in life at the age of around forty and which the carrier may transmit to his progeny. Senescence may perhaps be due to the accumulation of deleterious mutations, there are surely some, but this mechanism is not really documented, for the moment [17] (see Annex B).

Obviously, senescence is also determined by many *environmental factors* that constitute the basis of daily activity for a geriatrician. Human beings stand out from the other species because *Homo sapiens* is the only species which is able to control its own mean life span and which has witnessed a recent increase in this control. The reduction of our mortality was observed in every age category from new born to the elderly [1]. The human being is the only species whose life span increases after the reproduction phase "in disagreement with the conventional theories of senescence" [2, 6, 7].

8.2 Senescence and Inflammation

TIME magazine devoted several fully illustrated pages to inflammation and the role of inflammation in the pathophysiology of several chronic non-transmissible diseases, including rheumatoid arthritis, Alzheimer's disease and, above all, the clinical manifestations of atherosclerosis [18–20]. Inflammation, "the secret killer", states the editorial. Inflammation and the immune system are closely linked and depend on energy resources [21, 22] and there is much evidence that the inflammatory factors are, in a large part, produced by the adipose tissue [20, 23, 24].

The functional structures in charge of controlling the keys of the metabolism and the immune function have a common ancestor. For example, the adipose body of Drosophila, a fly familiar to every biologist contains same tissue structures that are comparable to the liver, immune and hematopoietic systems, and it is not surprising that these structures have evolved in parallel, in mammals. During evolution, in insects, the immune system has a receptor which is a protection against bacteria (through the liposaccharides of the bacterial wall), the Toll receptor, TLR, which activates a transcription factor, NF-kappa B, which is able to induce a metabolic cascade that synthesizes various mechanisms to stimulate defense against foreign invaders (virus, bacteria, parasites), i.e. the inflammatory cascade. At a certain moment in evolution, vertebrates attributed these mechanisms to two different tissues, the liver and the adipose tissue. Both preadipocytes and macrophages shared the same mesodermal origin, they differentiate early during embryogenesis following, in the first the hematopoietic lineage and in the second, the mesenchymal lineage.

High concentrations of macrophages in the adipose tissue of obese persons were firmly established a few years ago. Macrophages represent 5–10% of the cellular mass of the adipose tissue in normal individuals, this proportion increases to 65 in obese persons. The same result was observed in obesity of genetic origin and in experimental models of lipid induced overweight. In each case the adipose tissue is infiltrated by macrophages and a linear correlation was observed between the degree of obesity and inflammation biomarkers [23, 25].

Myriad pro-inflammatory signals either of endocrine origin or in relation with the lipid metabolism have been proposed and documented; cytokines and chemokines can interrupt insulin signaling and enhance glucagon signaling; the reverse is obtained with anti-inflammatory signaling [22]. The process is at the heart of the so-called immunometabolism, and varies from one individual to another. This is essential to the understanding and practice of personalized medicine. Geriatry does not escape from such a paradigm.

Macrophages originate from the medulla and their penetration of the adipose tissue is accompanied by an activation of the expression of chemotaxic genes such as the chemotactile cytokines and a factor of the complement precursor of C3a. Leptin, the adipostat hormone, also plays a role. From a histological point of view, macrophages and preadipocytes are very alike, but there are several specific markers which enable their identification. There are also gateways between the two groups of cells, from preadipocytes to macrophages, the differentiation being induced by the cytokines produced by the mature adipocytes. Macrophages have to eliminate all the external invaders by secreting several cytokines which are the basis of the immune response, they play a crucial role in the genesis of the atherosclerotic plaque as foam cells.

Insulin resistance is multi-factorial and precedes the appearance of diabetes. The excessive production of unesterified fatty acids by the adipose tissue participates in the loop formed by insulin which inhibits lipolysis [26]. The links with the inflammatory reaction are also well-documented: IL-6, the C-reactive protein, CRP, TNF-alpha, the sialic acid concentration, which are all biomarkers of the inflammatory reaction and are correlated with the appearance of type 2 diabetes. The correlation between CRP and insulin resistance, for example, is independent of the correlation between CRP and the incidence of coronary diseases. Still more convincing are the effects of high doses of aspirin which lower glycemia [27]. The inflammatory process risen from adipocytes is indeed one of the determinants of insulin resistance.

"Inflammageing" [28–31] is based on the observation that ageing and age linked chronic diseases were associated with a low level of inflammation with an elevation of several plasma markers [32, 33]. The various repeated stresses of our existence, including oxidative stress, would induce such a reaction. Such hypotheses still require full confirmation, we especially need a multicentric study with a big cohort using well-known, inflammatory markers such as CRP and therapeutic confirmation. The existence of inflammatory factors within the secretome of SCs is an argument favoring their role, at least, as an accelerator process. Nevertheless, one of the major arguments which can be opposed to the "ROS accumulation" hypothesis (first proposed by Harman in 1956, see [34]) is the existence in the organism of a large variety of buffers, which largely exceed the demand. Low level inflammation is only, for the moment, an attractive hypothesis which is only really documented in the clinical manifestations of atherosclerosis [34].

References

1. Swynghedauw B. L'homme malade de lui-même, Belin ed.; 2015.
2. Burger O. Human mortality improvement in evolutionary context. PNAS. 2012;109:18210–4.
3. Darwin CR. On the origin of species. London: John Murray; 1859.
4. Nesse RM, et al. Why we get sick. New York: Times Books; 1995.
5. Trevathan WR, et al., editors. Evolutionary medicine. New York: Oxford University Press; 1999. 480pp.
6. Flatt T. Plasticity of lifespan: a reaction norm perspective. Proc Nutr Soc. 2014;73:532–42.
7. Phelan JP, et al. Caloric restriction increases longevity substantially only when the reaction norm is steep. Biogerontology. 2006;7:161–4.
8. Alvergne A, et al. Evolutionary thinking in medicine. Cham: Springer; 2015.
9. Swynghedauw B, editor. Quand le gène est en conflit avec son environnement. Une introduction à la médecine darwinienne. Brussels: De Boeck; 2009.
10. Frelin C, et al. Biologie de l'évolution et médecine. Paris: Lavoisier; 2011.
11. Kirkwood TBL. Why do organisms age? In: Michel JP, et al., editors. Oxford text book of geriatric medicine, chap. 40, 3rd ed. Oxford: Oxford University Press; 2018.
12. Thomas H. Senescence, ageing and death of the whole plant. New Phytol. 2013;197:696–711.
13. Gems D, et al. Genetics of longevity in models organisms: debates and paradigms shifts. Annu Rev Physiol. 2013;75:621–44.
14. Jones OR, et al. Diversity of ageing across the tree of life. Nature. 2014;505:169–73.
15. Schultz MB, et al. When stem cells grow old: phenotype and mechanisms of stem cell aging. Development. 2016;143:3–14.
16. Wick G, et al. A darwinian-evolutionary concept of age-related diseases. Exp Gerontol. 2003;38:13–25.
17. Lemaitre JF, et al. Early-life trade-offs and the evolution of ageing in the wild. Proc R Soc B Biol Sci. 2015;282:209.
18. Gorman C, et al. The fires within. Time. 2004;163:44–51.
19. Steinberg D. Atherogenesis in perspective: hypercholesterolemia and inflammation as partners in crime. Nat Med. 2002;8:1211–7.
20. Weisberg SP, et al. Obesity is associated with macrophage accumulation in adipose tissue. J Clin Invest. 2003;112:1796–808.
21. Berg AH, et al. Adipose tissue, inflammation, and cardiovascular disease. Circ Res. 2005;96:939–49.
22. Hotamisligil GS. Inflammation, metaflammation and immunometabolic disorders. Nature. 2017;542:177–85.
23. Tchkonia T, et al. Cellular senescence and the senescent phenotype: therapeutic opportunities. J Clin Invest. 2013;123:966–72.
24. Wellen KE, et al. Obesity-induced inflammatory changes in adipose tissue. J Clin Invest. 2003;112:1785–8.
25. Xu H, et al. Chronic inflammation in fat plays a crucial role in the development of obesity-related insulin resistance. J Clin Invest. 2003;112:1821–183.

26. Swynghedauw B. Cholestérol, triglycérides et acides gras non estérifiés circulant chez 91 diabétiques. Le Diabète. 1968;16:40–4.
27. Woodward M, et al. A randomized comparison of the effects of aspirin and clopidogrel on thrombotic risk factors and C-reactive protein following myocardial infarction: the CADET trial. J Thromb Haemost. 2004;2:1934–40.
28. Campisi J, et al. Aging, cellular senescence, and cancer. Annu Rev Physiol. 2013;75:685–705.
29. Chung HY, et al. Molecular inflammation: underpinnings of aging and age-related diseases. Ageing Res Rev. 2009;8:18–30.
30. Freund A, et al. Inflammatory networks during cellular senescence: causes and consequences. Trends Mol Med. 2010;16:238–46.
31. Erusalimsky JD, et al. Mechanisms of endothelial senescence. Exp Physiol. 2008; 94(3):299–304.
32. Jurk D, et al. Chronic inflammation induces telomere dysfunction and accelerates ageing in mice. Nat Commun. 2014;2:1–13.
33. Olivieri F, et al. Circulating inflamma-miR in aging and age-related diseases. Front Genet. 2013;4:1–9.
34. Camici GG, et al. Molecular mechanism of endothelial and vascular aging: implications for cardiovascular disease. Eur Heart J. 2015;36:3392–403.

Conclusions

9

Abstract

For the moment, techniques for helping the elderly in their daily life are available and result in an improved health span. Globally, ageing is associated with a reduced capacity to adapt to environmental changes. One of the main obstacles to developing a general understanding of the senescence process is the making of ignorance developed by trendy spirits predicting immortality, thanks to magical senolytic therapies.

9.1 The Accession of Gerontechnologies

There are very likely as many theories on senescence as labs or groups working on the topic [1, 2]. Several have tried to simplify the problem, but this requires the setting aside of at least two major problems: the capacity to increase its own life span belongs to one unique living species, ours, and with ageing, the biology of human beings is far from simplified.

The new concept that has been developed, is not a new theory, but is based on convergent and solid experimental data that enable the establishment of a strong biological link between clinical ageing and cellular senescence. Such a thought is potentially rich for the future and we can imagine several biomarkers of senescence and possibly several new therapeutic approaches. Our life expectancy has increased by 2–3 months per year and seems to reach a plateau when it approaches the maximum life span of our species. Ageing in good health, if possible and if we are lucky enough, is facilitated *by* several very concrete advances, many of them have nothing to do with bench biology and belong to what we call gerontechnologies [3, 4]. Gerontechnology qualifies various technologies for helping old people and healthcare professionals and includes several technical advances that reduce social isolation (videophones, devices for calling emergency numbers), attenuate the loss of autonomy in daily life (such as orthopedic devices…) or cognitive disorders (such

© Springer Nature Switzerland AG 2019

B. Swynghedauw, *The Biology of Senescence*, Practical Issues in Geriatrics,
https://doi.org/10.1007/978-3-030-15111-9_9

as telemonitoring), and the installation of "smart homes". The positive effect of these measures has been frequently emphasized. Several papers have evidenced the improvement of the prognosis of a cancer (after 72 years [5]) or heart failure (after 80 years [6]), or, even, an Alzheimer's [7, 8] in patients having seriously adopted these sorts of technologies. These new growing technologies will certainly constitute one of the most important issues for the future of any health program [9].

9.2　　The Adaptive Capacities

Globally, ageing is associated with reduced ability to adapt to environmental changes, including stress and stress response, and a reduction of biological complexity (see Annex B). Cell proliferation is one of the responses of organisms to chronic stress and various aggressions. The progressive invasion of the human organism by SCs progressively reduces these adaptive capacities. A good example is the skeletal muscle which, normally in the young or adults, loses muscle cells during prolonged or strenuous exercise. During rest conditions, satellite cells (which are stem cells) are resynthesized and the previous potential is regenerated. Senescent skeletal muscle stem cells exhibit epigenetic alterations, which causes the aberrant expression of a gene, Hoxalpha 9. The ensuing consequence is the promotion of a pathway that results in a functional decline of the cell and the final result is a reduced number of satellite cells and a deficit in the total recovery of their initial potential. The clinical result is sarcopenia, a major problem in the elderly.

The story is the same for several other stem/progenitor cells, with important but different clinical consequences. It has been shown that the oscillatory properties of young cells, at least at the peripheral level, were modified and attenuated when cells were incubated in the presence of old serum. The attenuation of the circadian oscillations is another example of loss of adaptability with different biological mechanisms. With ageing, circadian oscillations are changed and attenuated. The biological rhythms are at the center of the adaptability of the organism.

One of the mechanisms of adaptation of an organ or organism is compensatory hypertrophy of the intact cells. In the case of senescence, young cells that still have intact regenerative capacities compensate for the loss of the organ cellular bank account by compensatory hypertrophy. Such a mechanism can easily be observed in the myocardium, but also in the kidney or the lungs, and could constitute an interesting, while imperfect, new target for therapy.

9.3　　The Gerontological Aspects of the Making of Ignorance

The "making of ignorance" is the title of a brilliant editorial of the review *Esprit* (July 2014) about the books of Robert Proctor and predictive medicine. Such a "making" also has an important geriatric dimension. In these times of transhumanism, we frequently hear trendy spirits predicting immortality in the near future or others proposing, more or less whacky, magic senolytic therapies, none of which have a solid scientific basis. Clearly, this does not mean that it is not possible to improve the daily life of the elderly and to increase health span to a time where ageing could be experienced under good conditions. These possibilities exist, but most of them are extremely expensive, which is the first and major problem for everyone interested in senotherapies for the future. The same arguments have been raised for cancer. In addition, these therapies are at an experimental stage and still require extensive approaches, especially on a clinical level [10, 11].

References

1. Swynghedauw B, et al. Le pourquoi du vieillissement. In: Artigou JY, et al., editors. Traité de cardiologie. SFC. Paris: Elsevier Masson; 2007. p. 1201–3.
2. Weinert BT, et al. Theories of ageing. J Appl Physiol. 2003;95:1706–16.
3. Rialle V. Technologies nouvelles susceptibles d'améliorer les pratiques gérontologiques. Rapport remis au Ministère de la Santé Mai 2000.
4. Ruellan du Crehu du Parc I. Les gérontechnologies: technologies nouvelles au service des personnes âgées de leurs aidants et des soignants. Université René Descartes Paris V. Cochin Paris. DIU formation à la fonction de médecin coordinateur d'Etablissement d'Hébergement pour Personnes Agées. Année 2010-2011. May be found on Internet.
5. Jonna S, et al. Geriatric assessment factors are associated with mortality after hospitalization in older adults with cancer. Support Care Cancer. 2016;24:4807–13.
6. Fleg JL. Exercise therapy for older heart failure patients. Heart Fail Clin. 2017;13:607–17.
7. Pimouguet C, et al. Benefits of occupational therapy in dementia patients: findings from a real-world observational study. J Alzheimers Dis. 2017;56:509–17.
8. Ménard J. Rapport Pour le malade et ses proches, chercher, soigner et prendre soin. Commission sur l'Alzheimer Novembre 2007.
9. Piau A, et al. Ageing society and gerontechnology: a solution for an independent living. J Nutr Health Aging. 2014;18:97–112.
10. Deursen van JM. The role of senescent cells in ageing. Nature. 2014;509:439–46.
11. Kirkland JL, et al. The clinical potential of senolytic drugs. J Am Geriatr Soc. 2017;65:2297–301.

Summary

10

Abstract

Maximum life span is an intangible genetic property of every living species, but human beings are unique as a living species in being able to control their mean life span. The present spectacular increase of human mean life span has radically transformed the world medical landscape. Transmissible diseases are no more the main cause of mortality and the chronic non-transmissible disease, appeared as the major source of morbi-mortality all over the world. A new concept has emerged which, although with some limitations, both clarified and simplified the view that we have of normal and pathological senescence. The concept is based on the central role of *CELLULAR SENESCENCE*.

Maximum life span is an intangible genetic property of every living species, but human beings are unique as a living species in being able to control their mean life span. The present spectacular increase of human mean life span has radically transformed the world medical landscape, including in developing countries. Transmissible diseases are no more the main cause of mortality and, recently (see the *GBD Study* in *Lancet* 2017), a new epidemiological group has been characterized, the chronic non-transmissible disease, which appeared as the major source of morbi-mortality all over the world. For years, the biology of senescence was considered as a complicated stochastic issue. Presently, based on the Hayflick seminal work, a new concept has emerged and has been developed mainly by the Mayo Clinic groups [1] which, although with some limitations, both clarified and simplified the view that we have of normal and pathological senescence. The concept is based on the central role of *CELLULAR SENESCENCE*.

The senescent cells, SCs, are characterized by an irreversible proliferation arrest of cells and can be identified by several biomarkers. Both the SC and its secretome are responsible for several physiological or pathological manifestations of ageing. A proof of concept, based on genetic manipulations in mice, was reported [2] and

© Springer Nature Switzerland AG 2019
B. Swynghedauw, *The Biology of Senescence*, Practical Issues in Geriatrics,
https://doi.org/10.1007/978-3-030-15111-9_10

confirmed by several groups. SCs were found in every human senescent organ. They are mainly generated by genome instability plus a hereditary component, telomere shortening, and epigenetic factors. The microbiota composition is also likely to be causally associated.

Proliferation arrest has functional consequences. The most important is located within the hypothalamus in which astrocytes play a major anti-ageing role. In skeletal muscle, ageing inhibits the regenerative capacity of satellite cells, the process also affects hair melanocytes, nephrons and tubules, chondrocytes, osteoblasts, several types of lung or liver cells, the beta Langerhans pancreatic cells, and the immune/hematopoietic system.

The insoluble (vesicles containing microRNAs) or soluble secretome participates in this autocrine activity. Extensive studies of SC secretome composition have been published. Secretomes are enriched in pro-inflammatory substances (the so-called "inflammageing"), several proteases and activators of cellular proliferations (potentially cancerogenic). Several others may play a role in the deregulation of circadian rhythms and in the frailty syndrome. The secretome of senescent epithelial cells also contains a number of carcinogenic substances and the senescent endothelial arterial cells are enriched in several atherogenic substances. There are also suggestions that the secretome of fibroblasts influences biological cycles.

To-day, the growing incidence of neurodegenerative diseases is a major public health problem, which is mainly linked to age through failures in proteostasis, but also to several environmental factors (pesticides). The heritability of AD and the role of inflammatory factors from the secretome have been evidenced, but, for the moment, the origin of this group is largely enigmatic. Ageing is associated with an increase in pulse pressure, arterial stiffness, a left ventricular impedance overload with LV hypertrophy, and a reduction in coronary reserve. Adult cardiocytes are SC and their reduction correlates with ageing and is associated with a compensatory hypertrophy of the remaining cells. Recently, several papers have suggested a role of proteostasis in the genesis of heart failure.

To a certain extent, contemporary human ageing proceeds against the evolutionary Darwin law. The remarkable plasticity of the human mean life span strongly suggests that environment plays a major role. Experimental findings have been proposed as a basis for a senotherapy. Nevertheless, major obstacle exists to any clinical applications, the first being the difficulty of suppressing SCs without producing any cancerogenic effect. For the moment the only validated therapies are caloric restrictions, physical exercise, and the gerontechnologies.

References

1. van Deursen JM. The role of senescent cells in ageing. Nature. 2014;509:439–46.
2. Baker DJ, et al. Naturally occurring p16Ink4a-positive cells shorten healthy lifespan. Nature. 2016;530:184–9.

Annex A: Senescence in Plants and Bacteria

Senescence belongs to life and exists in every living species. Plants belong to the tree of life and senesce just as other living species do. Nevertheless, this does not necessarily mean that the mechanisms of senescence are the same in every kingdom or even in every family of living species. A global theory of ageing is not possible, at least for the moment.

Plant senescence differs from animal senescence from many points of view: their longevity, from 10 to more than 2000 years, the role of telomere attrition and of hormonal status. There are plants that are reborn every year. Different experimental data has shown that several plants have a modular type mode of senescence (soy and spinach, for example) and that, globally, plant senescence being modular, the branches of a tree can senesce and die while the tree itself remains alive. In plants, senescence can be slowed by suppressing flowers or fruit. Such effects are local and the ablation of flowers in one branch has no effect on the others. Plants may be mono or dioecious. In plants, like in humans, females live longer than males. This observation gives weight to the argument that sees an environmental effect in these differences [1–4].

Senescence in *bacteria* is not easy to define or delineate and also poorly documented. The only specificity is the absence of any competition between reproduction and survival [5].

© Springer Nature Switzerland AG 2019
B. Swynghedauw, *The Biology of Senescence*, Practical Issues in Geriatrics,
https://doi.org/10.1007/978-3-030-15111-9

Annex B: Theories of Ageing

The following list is restricted to the other theories [6, 7] proposed in addition to the proposals from van Deursen, Childs, and others central to this work (see Figs. 3.1 and 4.1; Table B.1).

When we analyze these different hypotheses, what is sometimes surprising is the propensity of several authors to set out views that are more based on a philosophical than a scientific approach, and to limit their consideration to only a few aspects of senescence.

1. The disposable soma theory is a good example. The hypothesis presupposes that during evolution, living species, for purposes of reproduction, have to store and can store energy to maintain their "soma" and by so doing reduce all energy necessary for their existence and reproduction capacity, and consequently, shorten their life span. Such a view is in sharp contradiction with what can be

Table B.1 Main modifications observed during the general process of senescence, each gave rise to a theory of senescence

Evolutionary aspects
Accumulation of mutations [8]
Disposable soma theory [9]
Antagonistic pleiotropy theory [10]
Molecular aspects
Changes in the expression of genes regulating development and senescence
Catastrophic reduction in translation accuracy with formation of abnormal proteins
Somatic mutations with accumulation of DNA damage
Dys-differentiation
Cellular aspects
Programmed cell death by apoptosis
Replicative senescence and telomere attrition
Free radicals
The "wear-and-tear" hypothesis
Systemic aspects
Neuroendocrine senescence
Immunosenescence (stem cells decline) [11]
"Live fast, die young"
Hyperfunction theory: age is a quasi-programme [6]

© Springer Nature Switzerland AG 2019

B. Swynghedauw, *The Biology of Senescence*, Practical Issues in Geriatrics, https://doi.org/10.1007/978-3-030-15111-9

observed in human beings. It indeed would presuppose that a professional athlete would have a shorter life span than ordinary people, which contradicts the observation made by Antero-Jacquemin et al. [12].The life span of Olympic athletes is increased by about 7 years compared to the rest of the population.

2. The hyperfunction theory formulates the idea that the different processes responsible for growth and development are reactivated late in life and become responsible for hypertrophy and hyperplasia [13]. Such a theory does not account for the effects of the secretome.

3. The antagonistic pleiotropy hypothesis postulates that there are genes like those encoding the proteins of osteogenesis, which have beneficial effects in youth and deleterious effects in ageing. Several genes may be good candidates, but, for the moment, few have really been identified and there is no real demonstration that they have an effect on the reproductive capacity of an individual [10, 14].

Complexity: Is Senescence Linked to a Loss of the Complexity That Is Inherently Linked to Life?

The living systems are complex thermodynamically-open, dynamical, self-organized systems, which exchange energy and matter with an already complex environment. Lipsitz and Goldberger [15, 16] first proposed that ageing is characterized by a progressive loss of physiological complexity and a progressive impairment in the range of adaptive responses to the numerous stressors of the life. Such a view is supported by various observations made on circadian rhythms, respiratory dynamics, heart beats frequency, postural control, locomotor system, manual force production, brain networks... [16–18] (see also Annex E).

Annex C: Telomeres and Telomerase

In vertebrates, the DNA of the telomere is composed of a repetitive sequence of 6 bases enriched in guanosine, TTAGGG/CCCTAA. In humans, the length of this sequence is extremely variable (from 0.6 to 15 k pairs of bases), It is fairly easy to measure this DNA length and this has enabled several epidemiological studies [19–21]. Variability also exists between the chromosomes from one chromosome to another, and is, in part, heritable. Telomeres are associated with 17 proteins that regulate their accessibility (i.e., the fact that the telomere loop is opened or closed (Figs. C.1 and C.2). Telomerase is more an enzymatic complex than an ordinary enzyme. Telomerase is a reverse transcriptase capable of resynthesizing the

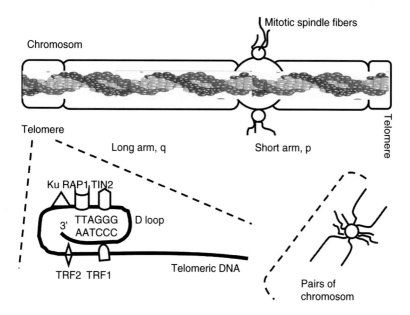

Fig. C.1 Telomere and telomerase structure. DNA itself is composed of two DNA strands. Chromosomes include the DNA strands themselves plus several proteins (histones) that permit translation. Telomeres are repetitive structures (the D loop, TTAGGG, and AATCCC) located at the two extremities of the chromosomic DNA. The telomerase is regulated by several proteins (Ku, RAP1, TIN2, TRF2, TRF1)

© Springer Nature Switzerland AG 2019
B. Swynghedauw, *The Biology of Senescence*, Practical Issues in Geriatrics,
https://doi.org/10.1007/978-3-030-15111-9

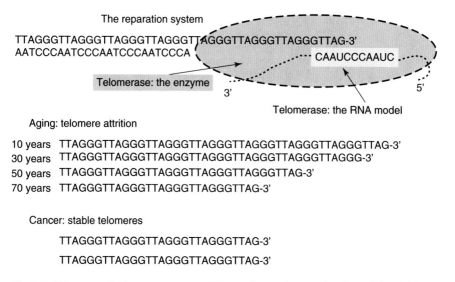

Aging: telomere attrition

10 years   TTAGGGTTAGGGTTAGGGTTAGGGTTAGGGTTAGGGTTAGGGTTAG-3'
30 years   TTAGGGTTAGGGTTAGGGTTAGGGTTAGGGTTAGGGTTAGGG-3'
50 years   TTAGGGTTAGGGTTAGGGTTAGGGTTAGGGTTAG-3'
70 years   TTAGGGTTAGGGTTAGGGTTAGGGTTAG-3'

Cancer: stable telomeres

TTAGGGTTAGGGTTAGGGTTAGGGTTAG-3'

TTAGGGTTAGGGTTAGGGTTAGGGTTAG-3'

Fig. C.2 Telomere and telomerase structure. Effects of age and cancer (see Sects. 3.3 and 6.1)

repetitive DNA structures from an RNA model. The structure of the integral human telomerase RNA subunit was recently reported [22].

The numerous levels of regulation vary from one cell to another and include a series of proteins, which, in turn, can be ribosylated, phosphorylated, or glycosylated... One of the important properties of telomeres is the capacity to emit salvage signals, such as p53, when the length of the telomeres reaches a critical minimal threshold. p53 itself can provoke a cellular response, which can be apoptosis or bring into play the senescent replicative process itself. Chronic inflammation is associated with ageing (see below Sect. 8.2). Chronic inflammation, as defined in experimental models using a few criteria, such as enlarged spleen, high systemic IL-6 and hepatic immune cell infiltration, can cause telomere dysfunction, in vitro and in vivo, because it is integrated in multiple positive feedback loops that may instigate oxidative stress [23].

In nature, there are many other solutions for resolving the same problem. Some viruses may utilize hairpin bed structures, specific transposable elements in certain insects. Our telomerase system is not unique (like the DNA structure!).

Annex D: MicroRNAs, miRs

miRs (they commonly are numbered) are small RNA sequences of ~22 nucleotides, noncoded and made by RNA genes [24–26]. They serve to block the transduction by specifically binding to complementary sequences located on the messenger RNAs, mRNA, (those that are used to translate the code into proteins). Several miRs are present in the plasma and, despite their fragility, they are potentially biomarkers utilizable in clinical practice. Other longer RNAs noncoding sequences exist and play a different regulatory role. It is important to emphasize that a given miR is not necessarily specific to a given mRNA, the specificity is for a complementary sequence of the mRNA and the same sequence can exist in two different mRNAs (see Sect. 3.5). miRs can be antagonized by "antagomirs", which are roughly their complementary sequences (Fig. D.1).

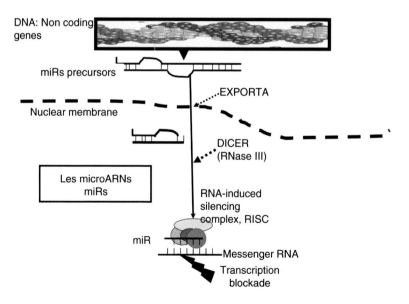

Fig. D.1 Synthesis of microRNAs. microRNAs precursor transcription is from the noncoding DNA and controls by EXPORTA to go through the nuclear membrane, and then process by an RNA-induced silencing complex, RISC. The blockade of the translation is due to a specific binding of the miR sequence to the corresponding messenger RNA sequence; this is why some miRs may inhibit several messenger RNAs

© Springer Nature Switzerland AG 2019
B. Swynghedauw, *The Biology of Senescence*, Practical Issues in Geriatrics,
https://doi.org/10.1007/978-3-030-15111-9

miR-21 regulates, in part, post-transcriptional processes. The regulation of collagen synthesis, for example, is mainly post-transcriptional [27]. miRs play a role in fetal reprogramming and in fibrogenesis in heart failure as shown by Thum [28, 29]. miRs are transported in microvesicles. A group of miRs (miR-55, 21 and 146a) is fairly specific of the inflammatory reaction (*inflamma miR*) [30].

Annex E: Circadian Rhythms, a Fundamental Basis of Life

Human genome sequencing led to an incredible explosion in every biological discipline, including physiology, defined as integrative biology, and, in addition to a complete rebirth of the discipline, it has contributed to the formation of a new vocabulary, new tools, new journals, new types of research and researchers. One of the first examples is the physiology and molecular biology of rhythms, which is so important in geriatric and cardiology. Rhythm physiology has literally been revolutionized by recent progress in genomics and by the publication of the diurnal transcriptome atlas in primates [31].

Rhythmicity is a very ancient property, in a large part linked to the light cycle, and which exists in every species, including plants. There are at least a circadian and a seasonal clock in plants [32] and bacteria [33]. These rhythms all have a genetic basis and, in humans, the so-called clock genes are expressed in nearly every tissue. The system is fully integrated and the peripheral clocks are synchronous with a central nervous clock system (Fig. E.1).

For the clinician, one of the most easy tools for exploring circadian variations is Holter monitoring of either the ECG or of arterial pressure [34]. Nevertheless, other biological rhythms exist, such as the daily variations of sleep and the menstrual cycle. Sleep disorders are one of the leading causes of consultation in geriatric. The analysis of biological rhythms has undergone recent major developments due to nonlinear analysis techniques and the introduction of the notion of chaos [35, 36], associated with the dawn of molecular technology [31].

The sleep/awake cycle exists in every animal species, and sleep deprivation is fatal and rhythmicity created by the sleep/awake alternation is a vital function. Biological oscillators integrate other oscillators and, for example, the sinusal heart rate integrates three other oscillators: a fast one, driven by respiration, a low-frequency oscillator, arterial pressure, and an ultra-slow monthly oscillator [36, 37]. Chaos is unlikely to cover the overall rhythm analysis, and for the heart rate, there is evidence that one can observe alternatively linear and nonlinear behavior of the rhythm [36, 38, 39]. Most of the circadian rhythms have an activity, which is reproducible from one individual to another and from one species to another. The dynamic of the oscillators is a complicated issue, which finally reaches a stable state. Heart rate, for example is, at rest, 70 beats/min, but it can reach 90–100 during exercise, but this is totally reversible and the heart rate at rest returns to 70. In the absence of pharmacological intervention, the two branches of the

© Springer Nature Switzerland AG 2019
B. Swynghedauw, *The Biology of Senescence*, Practical Issues in Geriatrics,
https://doi.org/10.1007/978-3-030-15111-9

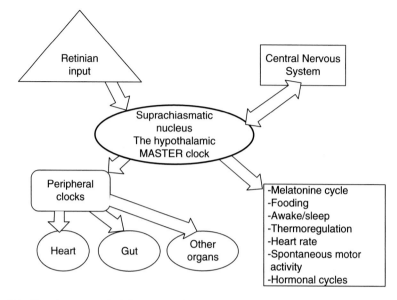

Fig. E.1 How the master clock is connected to peripheral clocks. Hypothalamic neurons receive light information by a direct retinohypothalamic tract and also some other information from the central nervous system. This information correct every day the central master clock phases which, in turn, will correct and adapt the slave peripheral clocks. Another synchronization occurs through eating, body temperature, and hormonal secretions. There are also suggestions that the SC secretome may modify clock operation (see Table 5.2)

autonomous system play a major and opposite role to control this system as a "push-pull mechanism", first described by Alberto Malliani [40].

From a more ideological point of view, it is tempting to say, as did Lipsitz [15], that life, health and youth are linked to complexity, to nonlinear, to chaotic behavior and that, conversely, illness, senescence and the approach of death, are accompanied by attenuated or irregular oscillations, meaning a dysregulation of our internal clocks. This is, for the moment, a declaration of principle, which requires factual confirmation. The frontier between stochastic and chaotic order is not self-evident, almost by definition, and we have to remember that chaotic behavior is defined as an organization with the appearance of disorder. Nevertheless, the hypothesis "is supported by observations showing an age related loss of complex variability in multiple physiologic processes" [15], while it can't be excluded that such a smoothing of these fluctuations may be a simple consequence of the decreased ability for exercise.

The Hypothalamic Clock

The circadian rotation of the earth has existed since the beginning of life and allows every living species to anticipate in the immediate future, the full content of the following day or night (eating, predator pressure, the sunrise for plants, the conditions of sleep), and not to react to these events. Nevertheless, as these clocks were fairly approximate, they have to be regularly set straight to be synchronous with the geophysical time. Many living species are transparent and can easily realign on daylight, but opaque species, like humans, require a fairly sophisticated system, which is connected to the optic nerve and receives the photonic influx. In the suprachiasmatic nucleus of the hypothalamus, there is a central master clock that controls the peripheral clocks located in every tissue [41] (Fig. E.1); this master clock regulates the phases of the peripheral clocks and their functions and is aligned on day/light through the retinal input [42, 43]. In addition, some axons are directly connected to the brain areas responsible for eating, of the sleep/awake cycle, and the melatonin/ ACTH secretions, which are linked to sleep [44]. Sleep, heart frequency, and body temperature are normally synchronous. Nevertheless, it is possible to disconnect these rhythms by specific lesions of the hypothalamus, and also during ageing.

The cell cycle duration is around a day and is under the control of a circadian clock, which regulates the expression of the different cyclins. The circadian clock is present both in each of the 20,000 neurons of the hypothalamic master clock and in every peripheral clock present in every organ. Molecular clocks are more or less the same everywhere. They are sensitive to hormones, energy availability, arterial pressure…. Biological clocks are equally present in living species in the absence of any central nervous system, like bacteria, cells in culture or plants [41].

Rhythmicity is a crucial property of life and as such it is extremely important that it is understood before "treating" or preventing the clinical consequences of senescence.

Molecular Mechanisms

The molecular basis of biological clocks is one of the oldest and most astonishing examples of what the Noble prize winner François Jacob [45] called "evolutionary tinkering". It results from a long, multifactorial evolutionary process, which started with the beginning of life. The molecular mechanism involves many genes, the rhythmic genes, and daily cycles in physiology are presumed to arise from their coordinated expression in every tissue [46]. In mice, 43% of all protein genes oscillate with a circadian rhythm. In primates, 81.7% of coding protein genes have a rhythmic expression with a quiescent period during early night. In particular, most of the ubiquitously expressed genes that participate in essential cellular functions exhibit rhythmic expression [31].

The molecular substrate of this clock and of cellular rhythmicity is well-documented [47–49]. It includes, at the transcriptional level, two retroactive loops, a negative one and a positive one, which both regulate the rhythmic variations of the concentrations of the key proteins that control the molecular clock (Fig. E.2). The basis of the system are the rhythmic variations of two transcription factors, CLOCK and BMAL1, that bind one to the other to form a heterodimer, which controls transcription

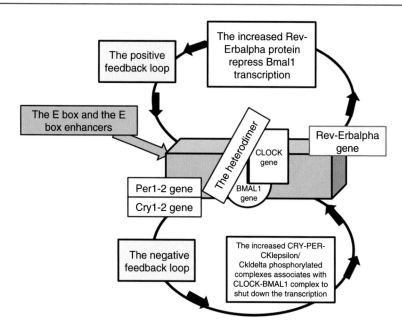

Fig. E.2 Molecular basis of the clock mechanism. It comprises two interactive feedback loops: a positive and a negative loop. The molecular basis of these biological clocks involves two loops, a negative and a positive loop, which control the concentrations of several proteins, which are key elements in the regulation of the physiological clocks. The heterodimer gene CLOCK/BMAL1 is responsible for the rhythmic transcription of five genes, mPer 1, 2 and 3 and mCry 1 and 2. The five proteins that are transcribed from these 5 genes enter into the nucleus to bind CLOCK/BMAL1, which results in a repression of their own transcription; this is the negative reaction loop. The positive reaction loop is also utilized by CLOCK/BMAL1. CLOCK/BMAL1 simultaneously activates the transcription of mRer and mCry and that of Rev-Erb alpha, a gene encoding REV-ERB alpha, which is a nuclear receptor which binds the Rev-Erb/ROR elements of the promotor of the transcription factor BMAL1 and by doing so, the transcription of this important regulator of the transcription. The final result is a decrease in the messengers RNA of mPer and the increase of mCry. When Per1 and mCry1 go into the nucleus to inhibit their own transcription, they simultaneously inhibit the transcription of Rev-Erbalpha and, by doing so, they activate the transcription of Bmal1. So, the two loops are co-regulated. The duration of a loop is around the dial, and is the duration of the period of the corresponding rhythm. These discoveries were recently completed by the publication by the Atlas of the gene of the circadian expression [31]. Furthermore, the heterodimer CLOCK/BMAL1 activates the periodic transcription of several genes, including the gene encoding vasopressin and several transcription factors that have an amplifying effect as for angiotensinogen

This system is essential for life and living species can't survive without it.[1] The cell cycle, which is the system controlling the production of mitoses and the activation of the cyclins, is also an oscillator with a period of around one hour (controlled by cyclins).[2]

---

[1] There are also several analogous systems like the system using the protein Timeless, TIM.

[2] In some species, this cycle is coupled with the circadian cycle [39].

The Peripheral Clocks

Obesity strongly attenuates the circadian variations of the Clock gene expression in the liver and adipose tissue and those of the adipose tissue hormones secretion as leptin or adiponectin.[3] The central and peripheral clocks regulate the expression of several transcription factors, including PPAR-alpha, which, in turn, regulates the expression of several metabolic genes. Plasma cholesterol, and also the levels of LDL, triglycerides and fibrinogen change significantly throughout the day. This has practical consequences, the chronotherapy and chronopharmacology. For example, because of the cyclic dependence of the HMG-CoA reductase, the effects of statins on plasma cholesterol are more pronounced if the drug is prescribed in the evening rather than in the morning.[4]

The Different Biological Rhythms: Sleep/Wakefulness; Hormones; Temperature

Sleep is under hypothalamic control and there is evidence that disruptions of the circadian rhythms parallels sleeping disorders and neuronal degeneration, indicating a progressive deterioration of the circadian pacemaker with ageing. Ageing does not always bring about changes in sleep quantity—in healthy ageing, the average sleeping time is around 6.5–7 h a day, but may cause changes in sleep architecture with increased night time restlessness and daytime sleepiness and a reduced amplitude of the sleep/awake rhythm (see, e.g., the Fig. 5 of Hofman [54] for the circadian rhythm in the number of arginine vasopressin-expressing neurons of the suprachiasmatic nucleus). For example, studies in young and elderly subjects under temporal isolation have reported a reduced amplitude and period of both body temperature and sleep/awake rhythms. This is accompanied by a change in the molecular responsiveness of the pacemaker to photic stimulation and a reduced expression of several genes encoding clock proteins [54].Nightly supplementation in melatonin was shown to improve sleeping disorders, suggesting a potential therapeutic role for this hormone.

The elderly presenting such sleep disorders appear at a greater risk of mortality. With advancing age, the circadian cycles start to be disrupted, which indicates a progressive deterioration of the circadian pacemaker regulation during ageing.

---

[3] Transgenic deletion in the genes controlling the circadian cycle such as Clock or Bmal1 reproduces the metabolic syndrome [47].

[4] Recently, a clock was identified in the myocardium [48–50]; this is an internal clock that does not depend on the autonomous nervous system and functions on an isolated coronary perfused heart. The messenger RNAs of BMAL1, CLOCK, Cry and Per were identified, and their expression varied in a circadian mode. In parallel, the expression of several metabolic genes varied during the day, with a peak at the beginning of the activity period (rats wake up in the evening). This is the case for GUT1 and 4 and mGS, which regulate glucose transport and glycogen anabolism, of the main enzymes in charge of the fatty acid catabolism and mitochondrial function and PPAR alpha. The variations are quantitatively important and some concentrations may double.

Obstructive sleep apnea increases in frequency with ageing, with prevalence rates as high as 60% above 60 years in certain meta-analyses. Involuntary, sometimes violent, movements may precede Parkinson's disease [54, 55].

Molecular Correlations

Globally, the heart, liver, gut and … the mind are at rest during the night. During the night, there is vagal activation and a sympathetic inactivation, sleep, bradycardia. Sleep exists in flies, and is essential for animal life. The two most popular theses state that either sleep is the time where brain protein synthesis is activated or that sleeping time is the moment when memory consolidates. Night and sleep time are in fact active periods of our life and the seat of an intense transcriptional activity. 10% of sequences are differentially expressed between night and day, while half of them are modulated by the daytime. There are cortical circadian genes whose expression is regulated by sleep alone, by sleep or by time only. Above all, there are as many genes that are activated during the nighttime than during the daytime, and they are not the same [56, 57].

In the peripheral area, the expression of 13% of genes differs very significantly between night and day. The expression of several constitutive genes (such as a gene regulating collagenase, an oxidase, several kinases) is cyclic with a period of 24 h plus two peaks, one in the daylight, the other during the night. Many gene expressions depend on light. There are some incomplete data suggesting that these dysregulations were associated with the progressive diminution of dreams during senescence [58].

Cell Physiology

Ageing is associated with a smoothing of most of the physiological rhythms, including the sleep/awake cycle, glycolysis, and calcium oscillations (see Sect. 5.4) [59–61]. Heart rate is not regular and its irregularities are consequences of factors affecting vasomotricity, rheology, and age. The variations of arteriolar motricity have chaotic behavior and under normal conditions, such a dynamic structure does not depend on pressure level since the correlation dimension remains unchanged at any level of cardiac flow, emphasizing that this property is an intrinsic property of the system. Conversely, the correlation dimension can be modified by pharmacological manipulations. There are systems, like the sinus heart rate, which, under normal conditions, function with a linear dynamic and may shift to chaotic behavior using a strange attractor [62].

Annex F: The Diabetic Heart

Diabetes is a well-documented risk factor, a risk for atherosclerosis; nevertheless, there is also a diabetic cardiomyopathy, DCM, directly linked to the development of diabetes both from a clinical and a pathophysiological view point, very likely linked to a diabetic microangiopathy (see also Sect. 6.3).

DCM is an entity occurring in type 1 or 2 diabetics, with normal coronary arteries, without any notion of alcoholism and with a normal arterial pressure. At the beginning, this is first a silencious diastolic dysfunctioning, mainly due to interstitial myocardial fibrosis and associated with cardiac hypertrophy. This is clearly not an ischemic cardiopathy of atherosclerosis origin in a diabetic. The first description is that from Rubler [63], although the 11 autopsies reported by Regan [64] 5 years later were much more convincing and demonstrate both the predominancy of myocardial fibrosis and the permeability of the coronary arteries [65–72]. This definition has been validated and accepted by cardiologists and diabetologists, including Braunwald in 1997 [73]; this is also the definition of the *Société Française de Cardiologie* [69]. DCM was also obtained in experimental model; the most complete review on the subject is from the group of Rayaz Malik [65].

From a clinical point of view, for a long time, DCM was considered as a rare disease. In fact, DCM is a frequent cause of heart failure. (1) 30% of hospitalized patients with heart failure are diabetics and diabetes is an important risk factor for heart failure (×2.4 in men, ×5.1 in women); nevertheless, these statistical values (Framingham, SHS, MESA, CHS and other trials) do not account for the multiple etiologies of heart failure in diabetes. (2) 12% of the type 2 diabetes are in heart failure and the annual incidence of heart failure is around 3.3%. In the UKPDS cohort, the prevalence of heart failure in type 2 diabetics is linked to HbA_{1C}, and for any 1% elevation of HbA_{1C}, the risk for heart failure increases by 8%. The risk correlates with the level of microangiopathy and especially with the kidney and ocular manifestations [74]. So, it is not surprising that diabetes was over-represented in the trials on heart failure (as SOLVD, ATLAS, V-HeFT or RESOLVD) and that insulin resistance or metabolic syndrome markers are good predictors of heart failure. (3) Several studies (Framingham, Tayside and Strong Heart Study) have evidenced a diastolic dysfunctioning in half of type 2 diabetics. Diastolic dysfunction is the first detectable functional abnormality witnessing DCM. (4) After myocardial infarction, 50% of diabetic patients may die within the following year. In addition, the

© Springer Nature Switzerland AG 2019
B. Swynghedauw, *The Biology of Senescence*, Practical Issues in Geriatrics,
https://doi.org/10.1007/978-3-030-15111-9

spectacular improvement in coronary mortality, which has been observed over the last 40 years does not concern diabetics [75]. In HFpEF, diabetes is twice as frequent as in controls. In coronary insufficiency, diabetes is associated with failure and in ischemic heart failure, the presence of diabetes is of bad prognosis. Such an adverse impact of diabetes suggests the presence of a latent DCM [71]. (5) For unknown reasons, arterial hypertension is significantly more frequent in diabetics. In the Strong Heart Study, it was to demonstrate that the filling pressure abnormalities in diabetes do not depend either on age or on arterial pressure. There are also other arguments suggesting the existence of a latent DCM, which may aggravate heart failure in diabetics [71]. (6) Diastolic dysfunction is very common in apparently healthy diabetics [76]. The systolic function is rarely normal both in experimental models and in humans [77].

From a Biological Point of View

By definition, DCM is not associated with changes in the large vessels and the most common alterations are interstitial fibrosis and arteriolar hyalinization [73].

The AMDCC Consortium recently succeeded in experimentally reproducing the human situation, i.e. a multifactorial situation that associates myocardial fibrosis with diabetes; this was obtained by a blockade of the leptin or the insulin pathways. Several papers proposed a unified theory to explain DCM [66, 67, 72]. Three cellular and metabolic abnormalities characterize DCM:

1. Hyperlipidemia is one of the leading causes of insulin resistance, but it may also be a cause of cardiac hypertrophy.
2. Systemic hyperinsulinemia can accentuate insulin action, such as in the myocardium, and be responsible for cardiac hypertrophy (summarized in [72]).
3. Hyperglycemia increases the production of superoxide ions and that of the "advanced glycation end-products", AGE.

Glossary

Coding part of the genome   the strand of DNA equivalent in sequence with the messenger RNA

Economy   economy can have different meanings. In this book, economy qualifies either the actual production of goods and services, more economic signifying more efficient, the production of one g of bread requiring less energy with this baker than with the other, or, using myothermal measurements in skeletal or cardiac muscle physiology, the number of ATP molecules burned or the oxygen consumption or the heat production per g of tension produced. A muscle contraction is more economic when it uses less energy to produce one g of tension [35, 78, 79).

Epigenetics   concerns a heritable phenotype that does not involve mutations, i.e. modifications in DNA sequence, but mostly changes in DNA methylation or histone modification. These changes modify gene expression without changing DNA sequence and last for several cell divisions. They play a role during development, growth, differentiation and senescence

Gene   unit of genetic information

MicroRNA (miR)   small regulatory RNA molecules, do not encode for a protein, block transcription at the mRNA level by specifically binding to a mRNA sequence (Annex D)

Noncoding DNA   roughly 95% of the genome; including the miRs precursors; the noncoding part of the genome includes many other regulatory elements

Retrotransposon   mobile elements in eucaryote genome present in high copy number that were active in the past and are now present as fossils in our genome. Can be reexpressed during senescence.

Transcription factor   protein that regulates gene expression by binding DNA in the control region of the gene

Transcriptome   the total RNA transcripts in the genome

Transcription   process in which information from DNA is converted into its RNA equivalent on the messenger RNA

Vernalization   a cold period, a long winter, which allows plants to accelerate their development in spring time; this is an epigenetic phenomenon.

© Springer Nature Switzerland AG 2019
B. Swynghedauw, *The Biology of Senescence*, Practical Issues in Geriatrics,
https://doi.org/10.1007/978-3-030-15111-9

References

1. Bondiansky R, et al. Sexual selection, sexual conflict and the evolution of ageing and lifespan. Funct Ecol. 2008;22:443–53.
2. Leopold AC, et al. Experimental modification of plant senescence. Plant Physiol. 1959;34:570–3.
3. Thomas H. Senescence, ageing and death of the whole plant. New Phytol. 2013;197:696–711.
4. Thomas H. Senescence. 2016. www.plantsenescence.org.
5. Nystrom T. Ageing in bacteria. Curr Opin Microbiol. 2002;5:596–601.
6. Falandry C, et al. Biology of cancer and aging: a complex association with the cellular senescence. J Clin Oncol. 2014;32:2604–11.
7. Weinert BT, et al. Theories of ageing. J Appl Physiol. 2003;95:1706–16.
8. Tomasetti C, et al. Stem cell divisions, somatic mutations, cancer etiology, and cancer prevention. Science. 2017;355:1330–4.
9. Kirkwood TBL. Evolution of ageing. Nature. 1977;270:301–4.
10. Leroi AM, et al. What evidence is there for the existence of individual genes with antagonistic pleiotropic effects? Mech Ageing Dev. 2005;126:421–9.
11. Schultz MB, et al. When stem cells grow old: phenotype and mechanisms of stem cell aging. Development. 2016;143:3–14.
12. Antero-Jacquemin J, et al. Mortality in female and male French Olympians: a 1948-2013 cohort. Am J Sports Med. 2015;43:1505.
13. Gems D, et al. Genetics of longevity in models organisms: debates and paradigms shifts. Annu Rev Physiol. 2013;75:621–44.
14. Giaimo S, et al. Is cellular senescence an example of antagonistic pleiotropy? Aging Cell. 2012;11:378–83.
15. Lipsitz LA, et al. Loss of "complexity" and aging. Potential applications of fractals and chaos theory to senescence. JAMA. 1992;267:1806–9.
16. Manor B, et al. Physiologic complexity and aging: implications for physical functionand rehabilitation. Prog Neuro-Psychopharmacol Biol Psychiatry. 2013;45:287–93.
17. Chatterjee A, et al. Aging and efficiency in living systems: complexity, adaptationa and self-organization. Mech Ageing Dev. 2017;163:2–7.
18. Goldberger AL, et al. What is physiologic complexity and how does it change with aging and disease? Neurobiol Aging. 2002;23:23–6.
19. Benetos A, et al. Short telomeres are associated with increased carotid atherosclerosis in hypertensive subjects. Hypertension. 2004;43:182–5.
20. Benetos A, et al. Short leukocyte telomere length precedes clinical expression of atherosclerosis. The blood-and-Muscle model. Circ Res. 2018;122:616–23.
21. Cherkas LF, et al. The effects of social status on biological ageing as measured by white-blood-cell telomere length. Aging Cell. 2006;5:361–5.
22. Nguyen THD, et al. Cryo-EM structure of substrate-bound human telomerase holoenzyme. Nature. 2018;557:190–5.

© Springer Nature Switzerland AG 2019

119

B. Swynghedauw, *The Biology of Senescence*, Practical Issues in Geriatrics,
https://doi.org/10.1007/978-3-030-15111-9

23. Jurk D, et al. Chronic inflammation induces telomere dysfunction and accelerates ageing in mice. Nat Commun. 2014;5:4172. https://doi.org/10.1038/ncomms5172.
24. Bartel DP. MicroRNAs genomics: biogenesis, mechanism and function. Cell. 2004;116:281–97.
25. Gewirtz AM. On future's doorstep: RNA interference and the pharmacopoeia of tomorrow. J Clin Invest. 2007;117:3612–3.
26. Großhans H, et al. The expanding world of small RNAs. Nature. 2008;451:414–6.
27. Besse S, et al. Nonsynchronous changes in myocardial collagen mRNA and protein during ageing: effect of Doca-salt hypertension. Am J Phys. 1994;267:H2237–44.
28. Thum T, et al. MicroRNAs in the human heart. A clue to foetal gene reprogramming in heart failure. Circulation. 2007;116:258–67.
29. Thum T, et al. MicroRNA-21 contributes to myocardial disease by stimulating MAP kinase signalling in fibroblasts. Nature. 2008;456:980–4.
30. Olivieri F, et al. Circulating inflamma-miR in ageing and age-related diseases. Front Genet. 2013;4:1–9.
31. Mure LS, et al. Diurnal transcriptome atlas of a primate across major neural and peripheral tissues. Science. 2018;359:eaao0318. https://doi.org/10.1126/science.AA0318.
32. Edwards KD, et al. Circadian clock components control daily growth activities by modulating cytokinin levels and cell division-associated gene expression in Populus trees. Plant Cell Environ. 2018;41:1468–82.
33. Bhadra U, et al. Evolution of circadian rhythms: from bacteria to humans. Sleep Med. 2017;35:49–61.
34. Carré F, et al. Spontaneously arrhythmias in a model of compensatory cardiac hypertrophy and in senescent rat: a Holter monitoring study. Cardiovasc Res. 1992;26:698–705.
35. Léger JJ, et al. From molecular to modular cardiology. How to interpret the million of data that came out from large scale analysis of gene expression? Arch Mal Coeur Vaiss. 2006;99:231–6.
36. Jasson S, et al. Instant power spectrum analysis of heart rate variability during orthostatic tilt using a time-frequency domain method. Circulation. 1997;96:3521–6.
37. Mansier P, et al. Linear and non-linear analysis of heart rate variability: a minireview. Cardiovasc Res. 1996;31:371–9.
38. Berger P, et al., editors. Des rythmes au chaos. Paris: Odile Jacob Sciences; 1994.
39. Elbert T, et al. Chaos and physiology: deterministic chaos in excitable cell assemblies. Physiol Rev. 1994;74:1–47.
40. Malliani A. Principles of cardiovascular neural regulation in health and disease. Boston: Kluwer Acad Pub; 2000.
41. Schibler U, et al. A web of circadian pacemakers. Cell. 2002;111:919–22.
42. Buijs RM, et al. Circadian and seasonable rhythms. The biological clock tunes the organs of the body: timing by hormones and the autonomic nervous system. J Endocrinol. 2003;177:17–26.
43. Saper CB, et al. The hypothalamic integrator for circadian rhythms. Trends Neurosc. 2005;28:152–7.
44. Touitou Y. Human ageing and melatonin. Clinical relevance. Exp Gerontol. 2001;36:1083–100.
45. Jacob F. Evolution and tinkering. Science. 1977;196:1161–6.
46. Zhang R, et al. A circadian gene expression atlas in mammals: implications for biology and medicine. Proc Natl Acad Sci U S A. 2014;111:16219–24.
47. Hatanaka F, et al. Keeping the rhythm while changing the lyrics: circadian biology in ageing. Cell. 2017;170:599–600.
48. Reppert SM, et al. Coordination of circadian timing in mammals. Nature. 2002;418:935–41.
49. Sato TK, et al. A functional strategy reveals Rora as a component of the mammalian circadian clock. Neuron. 2004;43:527–37.
50. Staels B. When the clock stops ticking, metabolic syndrome explodes. Nat Med. 2006;12:54–5.
51. Portman MA. Molecular mechanisms and circadian rhythms intrinsic to the heart. Circ Res. 2001;89:1084–6.
52. Young M, et al. Clock genes in the heart: characterization and attenuation in hypertrophy. Circ Res. 2001;88:1142–50.

53. Young ME, et al. Intrinsic diurnal variations in cardiac metabolism and contractile function. Circ Res. 2001;89:1199–208.
54. Hofman MA, et al. Living with the clock: the circadian pacemaker in older people. Ageing Res Rev. 2006;5:33–51.
55. Sterniczuk R, et al. Sleep disturbances in older ICU patients. Clin Interv Aging. 2014;9:969–77.
56. Cirelli C, et al. Extensive and divergent effects of sleep and wakefulness on brain gene expresson. Neuron. 2004;41:35–43.
57. Martino T, et al. Day/night rhythms in gene expression of the normal murine heart. J Mol Med. 2004;82:256–64.
58. Guénolé F, et al. Le rêve au cours du vieillissement normal et pathologique. Psychol Neuropsychiatr Vieil. 2010;8:87–96.
59. Goldbeter A. Biochemical oscillations and cellular rhythms. The molecular bases of periodic and chaotic behaviour. Cambridge: Cambridge University Press; 1996.
60. Pagani I, et al. Serum factor in older individuals change cellular clock properties. Proc Natl Acad Sci U S A. 2011;108:7218–23.
61. Touitou Y, et al. Modifications of circadian and circannual rhytthms with ageing. Exp Gerontol. 1997;32:603–14.
62. LePape G, et al. Statistical analysis of sequences of cardiac interbeat intervals does not support the chaos hypothesis. J Theor Biol. 1997;184:123–31.
63. Rubler S, et al. New type of cardiomyopathy associated with diabetic glomerulosclerosis. Am J Cardiol. 1972;30:595–602.
64. Regan TJ, et al. Evidence for cardiomyopathy in familial diabetes mellitus. J Clin Invest. 1977;60:885–99.
65. Asghar O, et al. Diabetic cardiomyopathy. Clin Sci. 2009;116:741–60.
66. Bell DSH. Diabetic cardiomyopathy. Diabetes Care. 2003;26:2949–51.
67. Bell DSH. Heart failure. The frequent, forgotten and often fatal complication of diabetes. Diabetes Care. 2003;26:2433–41.
68. Boudin S, et al. Diabetic cardiomyopathy revisited. Circulation. 2007;115:3213–23.
69. Charniot JC, et al. Coeur et diabète. In: Cardiologie et maladies vasculaires. SFC ed. Paris: Masson; 2007. p. 1206–9.
70. Lavis VR, et al. Endocrine disorders and the heart. In: Willerson JT, Cohn JN, editors. Cardiovascular medicine. 2nd ed. New York: Churchill Livingstone; 2000. p. 1921–5.
71. Marwick TH. Diabetic heart diseases. Heart. 2006;92:296–300.
72. Poornima IG, et al. Diabetic cardio-myopathy. The search for a unifying hypothesis. Circ Res. 2006;98:596–605.
73. Williams GH, et al. The heart in endocrine and nutritional disorders. In Braunwald E, editor. Heart disease, chap. 61, 5th ed. Philadelphia: Saunders WB; 1997. p. 1902–5.
74. Cheung N, et al. Diabetic retinopathy and risk of heart failure. J Am Coll Cardiol. 2008;51:1573–8.
75. Haffner SM. Coronary artery disease in patients with diabetes. N Engl J Med. 2000;342:1040–2.
76. Zabalgoita M, et al. Prevalence of diastolic dysfunction in normotensive, asymptomatic patients with well-controlled type 2 diabetes. Am J Cardiol. 2001;87:320–3.
77. Vinereanu D, et al. Subclinical LV dysfunction in asymptomatic patients with type 2 diabetes, related to serum lipids and glycated hemoglobin. Clin Sci. 2003;105:591–9.
78. Alpert NR, Hamrell BB, Mulieri LB. Heart muscle mechanics. Ann Rev Physiol. 1979;41:521–37.
79. Swynghedauw B. Molecular mechanisms of myocardial remodeling. Physiol Rev. 1999;79:215–62.

Printed in the United States
By Bookmasters